Treatment for Body-Focused Repetitive Behaviors

"*Treatment for Body-Focused Repetitive Behaviors: An Integrative Psychodynamic Approach* offers clarity, guidance, and hope. Nakell possesses a deep understanding of this difficult issue, and how fortunate for suffering individuals – and the therapists who treat them – that this resource is now available to them."

B. Natterson-Horowitz, *MD, Harvard Medical School*

"Nakell provides outstanding guidance to psychotherapists who want to engage in deep work while promoting behavioral change with a focus on translating body language into words to heal both physical and psychological scars. Her integrative, psychodynamic approach is powerful and extremely clinically relevant; this book is an important contribution to our field."

Molyn Leszcz, *MD, FRCPC, CGP, DFAGPA,*
professor of psychiatry, University of Toronto, and president,
the American Group Psychotherapy Association

"Nakell effectively outlines what is currently known about BFRBDs, the history of BFRBD treatment, and gaps in the current literature. Her utilization of case studies to illuminate how to engage in psychodynamic treatment with this population is unique and distinguished. I will certainly use this book in my course on the subject."

Mohammad Jafferany, *MD, FAPA, MCPS (Derm.),*
clinical professor of psychiatry and psychodermatology,
Central Michigan University, and executive secretary,
Association for Psychocutaneous Medicine of North America

Treatment for Body-Focused Repetitive Behaviors is the first book to establish the theory and practice of a psychodynamic approach to treating body-focused repetitive behavior disorders (BFRBDs), such as hair pulling, skin picking, and cheek, lip and cuticle biting. Chapters set out a new framework for understanding and treating BFRBDs, one grounded in attachment theory and neurobiological research.

Stacy K. Nakell is a licensed clinical social worker, certified group psychotherapist and certified clinical trauma professional. She provides psychotherapy to people struggling with body-focused repetitive behaviors and provides clinical consultation.

Routledge Focus on Mental Health

Routledge Focus on Mental Health presents short books on current topics, linking in with cutting-edge research and practice.

Titles in the series

For a full list of titles in this series, please visit www.routledge.com/Routledge-Focus-on-Mental-Health/book-series/RFMH

Treatment for Body-Focused Repetitive Behaviors
An Integrative Psychodynamic Approach

Stacy K. Nakell

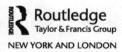

Routledge
Taylor & Francis Group

NEW YORK AND LONDON

First published 2023
by Routledge
605 Third Avenue, New York, NY 10158

and by Routledge
4 Park Square, Milton Park, Abingdon, Oxon, OX14 4RN

Routledge is an imprint of the Taylor & Francis Group, an informa business

Library of Congress Cataloging-in-Publication Data
Names: Nakell, Stacy K., author.
Title: Treatment for body-focused repetitive behaviors : an integrative
    psychodynamic approach/Stacy K. Nakell.
Other titles: Routledge focus on mental health.
Description: New York, NY : Routledge, 2023. | Series: Routledge focus
    on mental health | Includes bibliographical references and index.
Identifiers: LCCN 2022016369 (print) | LCCN 2022016370 (ebook) |
    ISBN 9781032284880 (hardback) | ISBN 9781032289144 (paperback) |
    ISBN 9781003299097 (ebook) Subjects: MESH: Disruptive, Impulse
    Control, and Conduct Disorders—therapy | Self-Injurious Behavior—
    therapy | Psychotherapy, Psychodynamic—methods
Classification: LCC RC480.5 (print) | LCC RC480.5 (ebook) | NLM WM
    192 | DDC 616.89/14—dc23/eng/20220510 LC record available at
    https://lccn.loc.gov/2022016369
LC ebook record available at https://lccn.loc.gov/2022016370

ISBN: 978-1-032-28488-0 (hbk)
ISBN: 978-1-032-28914-4 (pbk)
ISBN: 978-1-003-29909-7 (ebk)

DOI: 10.4324/9781003299097

Typeset in Times New Roman
by Apex CoVantage, LLC

Contents

Acknowledgments

As a healer, I would like to acknowledge the roots of my training in unacknowledged ancestral wisdom. This includes my own determined ancestors who forged a path as Jews from Poland and Russia to the United States and whose progeny number a great many psychotherapists. I also want to honor the indigenous roots of group psychotherapy in the format of the group circle, traditionally around a fire. I want to thank Joseph LePage for my training in 1996 in Integrative Yoga Therapy and also to acknowledge the deep Indian roots of that practice. It is by connecting to the wisdom of my body, my community and the earth that I hold space for growth for those I treat, and I am humbled by this opportunity to add my own wisdom to the collective healing space.

I would like to give a special thanks to Publisher Anna Moore for recognizing the value of my voice. She has enabled me to share my unique approach to BFRB treatment with the wider community of mental health care professionals, bringing this project from query to reality in less than a year. I am honored to share my work in this Routledge Focus series.

Many thanks to Dr. Molyn Leszcz, Dr. Mohammad Jafferany, and Dr. Barbara Natterson-Horowitz for their generosity in reading this manuscript and supporting me through this journey toward publication. I am so touched by how each has believed in me and lifted me up.

I couldn't have made it to this point without my dear writing coach/friend Cecily Sailer. Our relationship began in 2011, and she has always inspired within me the faith that if I kept writing this book even when I felt like giving up I would one day meet this very goal.

Thank you to my friends and colleagues who provided editing and emotional support, including Gabi Snyder, Jessica Burroughs, Teri Schroeder, Dr. Lavanya Shankar, Luce Fuller, Gianna Viola, Dr. Richard Holt, Jeanne Bunker, Dr. Jan Morris, Dr. Suzanne Phillips, Dr. Carlos Canales and Dr. Shelby Weltz, and to Kelly McGettigan, Brooke Robb and Dr. Neisha Hootman for research assistance.

I am so grateful for the contributions from the clients you will meet in these chapters. Each gave me permission to publish the vignettes under pseudonyms after assessing them to be accurate and reflective of their experiences with me in therapy.

I am also grateful to the *International Journal of Group Psychotherapy*, for granting me permission to share portions of case studies I featured in the 2015 short report, "A Healing Herd: Benefits of a Psychodynamic Group Approach in Treating Body-Focused Repetitive Behaviors." © The American Group Psychotherapy Association reprinted by permission of Taylor & Francis Ltd, www.tandfonline.com on behalf of The American Group Psychotherapy Association.

The case study "Colt" in Chapter 8 was featured in 2021, in "Psychodynamic Approach in the Treatment of Trichotillomania" in *Deermatologic Therapy* through John Wiley & Sons, Inc.

And last, but certainly not least, I would like to thank Lynne Monkarsh Nakell, Jessica Nakell Burroughs, Douglas Lee Holloway, Donald "Pops" Billingsley, Hollee Holloway, Samantha Lee Farr and Maysie Camille Hogue for teaching me most of what I know about secure attachment.

Introduction

If you are a therapist, you may not even remember hearing of hair pulling, or trichotillomania, in your diagnosis class in graduate school. Or you may have learned, in school or in professional trainings, that this disorder is easily solvable through behavioral change. You may notice your clients fidgeting a lot during sessions and feel at a loss for how to address this, or even whether it is appropriate to mention it at all. You may have found this book by googling "trichotillomania" after a client asked for your help with it.

If so, I was right there in your shoes in the spring of 2002, when I first googled "hair pulling" and entered into what would become the abiding passion of my career. At the time, I was working as counseling director at a teen center for LGBTQIA+ youth. I was spreading the word about an 8-week group I was forming (my first solo group) for those who wanted to work on self-harming behaviors, and a teen, Iris, came to my office to ask, "I pull out my hair. Do I qualify for your group?" I knew enough to accept her. "Of course, please join. The group is for anyone who wants to find ways to be nicer to themselves," I told her. But as soon as she left, I had to look it up!

At that time, trichotillomania was a little-known disorder and there was no information to be found about skin picking.

DOI: 10.4324/9781003299097-1

I found most of the available information through the Trichotillomania Learning Center (now the TLC Foundation for BFRBs) website, which has provided resources to those struggling with body-focused repetitive behaviors such as hair pulling since its founding in 1990, and, later, for those struggling with skin picking and cheek biting. I found some information about the course and consequences of BFRBDs but not a lot about their etiology or function. The only recommended treatment option was cognitive and behavioral treatment, including habit reversal therapy.

Iris did join the group. The issues she brought to the table were in the same vein as the issues of those who were cutting themselves – the underlying relational ruptures, low self-esteem and negative behaviors fueling self-hate – though they had a different flavor, even more secretive, accompanied by even more shame. And I noticed that Iris's amiability was in contrast to the outward anger and irritability of those in the group who were engaging in cutting. Members of the group talked through some of their similarities and differences.

The group helped Iris detoxify from the shame of pulling out her eyelashes. After the group ended, I saw her weekly, individually, for around 6 months, and we followed the trail of her hair-pulling history. We traced the first pulled eyelashes to a difficult math class right in the middle of her parents' divorce. We also noticed that the behaviors increased at times of relational stress and lessened when she felt safe in relationships.

By the time Iris left the teen center, she had been able to reduce her reliance on hair pulling. I was delighted when, last year, 20 years after our work ended, she contacted me to let me know that our early work had been foundational for her, that she had continued therapy and continued to find healthier relationships. She showed me photos of her wife and told me that hair pulling was no longer a coping strategy.

My claim to expertise in helping those who struggle with picking, pulling and biting is this: over the past 2 decades of working with this population, my clients usually – in fact, almost always – get better over time. They get better not only at managing their body-focused repetitive behaviors but also at regulating painful emotions. They become more assertive in relationships, develop healthier connections and are more inclined to share their feelings with others, enhancing their quality of life.

In the tradition of heuristic research, I have immersed myself in the study of BFRBDs and their treatment. Moustakas (1990) explains the importance of this immersion,

> Once the question is discovered and its terms defined and clarified, the researcher lives the question in waking, sleeping, and even dream states . . . The immersion process enables the researcher to come to be

on intimate terms with the question – to live it and grow in knowledge and understanding of it.

(p. 27)

Along the way, I have learned a great deal about how these behaviors both provide deep comfort and lead to terrible isolation.

If we understand picking and pulling as a sign of a psychic wound of some sort, we can follow the path of the disorder like a line of breadcrumbs to enable deeper healing. Reviewing the psychosocial context of some pivotal moments, like the first hairs pulled or a moment when the picking got very intense, I can help my clients to articulate the stories of their lives. The telling and witnessing of these stories reveal the complexities of the client's unique relationship with skin picking or hair pulling. And then, voilà, the behaviors may slowly loosen their grip!

The therapeutic relationship is where the magic happens. Being aware of the transference, where clients unconsciously project their attachment figures onto me, and my countertransferential reaction to these projections are key to this relational interplay. I learn most of what I need to know about my clients' attachment disruptions from my experience being in the room with them.

When we sit together with somatic awareness, I can help clients restart whatever pieces of emotional regulation process may have been hijacked along the way. My nervous system can help their nervous systems get that precious experience of being able to relax, fully, under the holding gaze of the (m)other. As I help them shake off shame and calm them and listen to them when they are sad or angry or hopeless, we can create new neural pathways for those feelings to be acceptable. A good therapeutic alliance can create an earned secure attachment. It is never too late!

From this lens, the whole point of treatment is to go beneath the surface of psychic wounds to get to their root. And, in this case, with the dermis – consisting of hair, skin and nails – being the literal site of the behavior at hand, don't we have to go below the surface to see what is motivating the restless hands of pickers and pullers?

If you are someone who likes to find the easiest answer to problems, who likes to focus on fixing symptoms rather than helping clients heal at a deeper level, this book is probably not for you. On the other hand, if you are interested in truly understanding the complexities and unique functions of these behaviors, and in the potential of the therapeutic relationship to heal them, you have come to the right place.

Some of the most powerful words you will read are those of clients. I am so grateful for their informed consent for me to include elements of their treatment in this work and as well as their participation in post-treatment interviews, conducted by independent research assistants. Each client picked a pseudonym and had an opportunity to read and give feedback on these studies prior to publication. In some cases, as noted, stories from similar clients are woven together into one.

One day a member of my therapy group, about whom I have written and presented, with his consent, expressed some annoyance that I was asking him to be vulnerable for my book. He wondered why I never had to be vulnerable in return. I took that as a welcome challenge to consider the potential benefits of being more transparent about my own history with skin picking.

In a meta-analysis of the literature, Hill et al. (2018) found that effective therapist self-disclosure can facilitate client exploration, foster understanding and lead to better functioning, providing a sense of universality to counter isolation. I have shared my history with skin picking with a number of clients, particularly to help them feel less alone in their struggles and to shake off shame. The authors note that therapist self-disclosure must be congruent with client needs and should be used sparingly and deliberately.

When I first worked with Iris, I had no idea that skin picking and trichotillomania were connected, or why I was so drawn to help her. It took a year or two for me to connect the dots. At about the same time the mental health field began to make the connection too, and skin picking has now become part of the BFRB conversation. Since then, my own decades-long relationship with skin picking has been my case study #1 for understanding the complex roots of body-focused behaviors. When I was at the worst of my skin picking, the disorder interfered with my self-esteem and my social, work and romantic lives. I would have rated it a 10 on the distress scale.

After recovering from an eating disorder, I had worked with adults battling anorexia, bulimia and binge-eating disorder for several years. I had seen that a psychodynamic approach was the key to resolving behavioral issues on a deep and sustaining level. In 2009, I attended a 3-day ComB workshop with its founder Dr. Mansueto and was clear that this behavioral approach focused on resolving symptoms was not going to be a fit for me. I wasn't looking for a quick fix; I was seeking to understand the connection between my comorbid conditions of depression, anxiety, body dysmorphic disorder and post-traumatic stress disorder (PTSD) and my chronic and destructive skin picking. Without a template for a psychodynamic approach to body-focused behaviors, I had to chart my own course.

Case study #1

In 2016, I was fortunate to be invited into a group of women therapists, founded by Dr. Jan Morris, whose mission was to explore the relationship between our experiences as female-identified group therapists, our relationship to our own aggression and the impact of gender dynamics on our countertransference work with clients. Dr. Morris and my longtime consultant, Jeanne Bunker, modeled the healthy disclosure of their own exploration of this topic on our panel at the American Group Psychotherapy Association's AGPAConnect in 2018, and in chapters in the 2021 book *Women, Intersectionality and Power in Group Therapy Leadership.*

Each has mentored me in expressing my unique voice. Bunker (2021) acknowledged the need for women to harness their power in order to overcome cultural obstacles, noting, "Ambition is an integration of desire, aggression and bravery" (p. 137). Over two decades of work together she helped me to harness my desire and aggression toward my goal of adding my voice to the literature. Dr. Morris helped me to understand that excavating my own curdled aggressive energy would be key to helping my clients externalize theirs. Morris (2021) explains, "Two key factors in working effectively with aggression in groups are the female therapist's comfort with her internal experience of aggression as well as her ability to tolerate aggression coming at her" (p. 121).

By the time I presented my autobiographical paper "White Lightning" at the inaugural panel of *Women and Aggression: History, Healing and Power* at the 2018 American Group Psychotherapy Association (AGPA)Connect meeting, I had almost completely stopped picking my skin. Telling my story quite literally did lead me into remission, which in turn has led to long-term recovery. To this day, I continue to engage only in healthy, though very enjoyable, grooming rituals, such as plucking unwanted hairs from my chin. Yes, I said it! We all do it! And I always keep putty or other sensory tools at the ready. My hands, when restless, are engaged in healthier pursuits.

I have decided that the benefits of being transparent warranted sharing parts of this previously unpublished paper with you all. In doing so, I am hoping to model the healthy disclosure of a body-focused behavior I once found shameful. I hope that this story will illuminate for therapists how depth work, while painful, and slow, can lead to integration of hated parts of the self and, ultimately, a new relationship with the skin and the self.

White Lightning

My personal experience of discovering skin picking as a primary coping mechanism was a confluence between a teenage acne outbreak, a lack of social skills and a fragile sense of self. When I learned from my mother that she experienced chronic hives during the first 2 years of my life, as she coped with two small children and a troubled marriage, I felt deep sadness. Her skin, my skin, had always been somehow connected, and now I had a story on which to weave my understanding.

My relationship with my father embodied generations of deeply strained parent/child relationships, with the silent treatment a deadly force for my blossoming assertive needs. I learned from an early age that my anger was unwelcome to him, and as a result I swallowed copious amounts of rage. In the sixth and seventh grades, I lost my two most positive attachment figures, my Grandpa Bill and my dog, Tarheel, and my rage turned into deep depression. I was terribly socially awkward, desperate for attention and vulnerable to abuse from male peers and others. I often reflected on how much I hated my unruly wavy hair and I could never figure out the right clothes to wear. Everything was all wrong.

And I picked my skin. I had always been fidgety and uncomfortable in my skin. Once I hit puberty, I found that picking at pimples on my face gave me something to do with my hands, while at the same time making me look as ugly as I felt. My body's thwarted need to express rage found an outlet in my hands, and my lifelong relationship with skin picking began.

I hated the acne on my face. After visiting my first dermatologist, an acne medication I tried led to disgusting green pustules for over a week. The green pus symbolized something that felt true about me as I rode on the bus, alone, avoiding eye contact. I was unacceptable and I needed to hide. For me, skin picking became both a shield and a self-directed sword.

By the seventh grade, I was experiencing a manifestation of what I describe in Chapter 2 as holes in my psychic skin. I simply did not have a sense of self, and that feeling was raw and shameful. Sometimes, at the worst moments, I could feel my skin ache all over. I covered up this horrible flaw as best I could. I had perfect grades and good relationships with teachers, but my peers could sniff it out – my lack of skin, my insecurity. I never could figure out how to belong and I was filled with despair, even though I was trying my very best.

In my late twenties, once I let go of my eating disorder, my skin picking became more violent. I discovered that when I got too full of frustration I could go into the bathroom, look in the mirror, and pick and pick and pick, until there was nothing more to pick. I would experience an amazing sense of relief. I could lose hours in that feeling, until emerging and taking stock of the red bumps on my face would lead me deeper into self-hate. I desperately needed an outward, physical release of all the aggression I was turning on myself. I think my life depended on meeting that need.

Thankfully, by my early thirties I had found three outlets for my frustration: therapy, writing and boxing. My therapist, a male, was able to effectively meet my aggression both firmly and with compassion. He picked up on my history as a scapegoat. When I was preparing to join his therapy group, he was clear about wanting me to lean on him for help with early group interactions. I sat next to him during each session, checking in with him about how much and what to share about myself and my reactions to others. In this way, he was able to help me avoid the tendencies that might lead me back into that familiar role.

At around the same time, I followed the trail that had taken root for me in 1984, when I attended the semi-finals of boxing in the Olympics. This pursuit led me to the Austin Women's Boxing Club. Coach Julia Gschwind introduced me to the healthy sublimation of aggression, as she prepared me for an amateur fight in the master's division. My ring name, White Lightning.

Julia is a third-degree black belt in Kajukimbo, an art that embodies the concepts of respect for one's opponents, teammates, coaches and self. These same concepts underlie all activities at her gym and provided a background for me to grow into my own power. I grew more at ease as I watched Julia's mastery of her own aggression, letting it out in doses as needed to set boundaries but never to retaliate or control.

She taught me to listen to my inner self for guidance rather than look to her as my ultimate authority. Sparring sessions between Julia and me were infrequent but epic as I prepared for my fight, as we share a similar primal resistance to being backed into a corner. We sparred with intensity, focus and respect for each other's strength and skills, literally matching each other's aggression, with both of us exiting the ring bruised and triumphant, two females still standing. We now coach a women's team together.

Boxing helped me to release layers and layers of aggressive energy that had been stored up in my body. Writing about my relationship with aggression helped me metabolize it, make sense of it and work with it. I came to understand that when anger isn't expressed, it has to go somewhere. If it is turned inward, it becomes a force of aggressive energy. For me, skin picking was largely an expression of this energy building up, and being let out, bit by bit. Many of my feelings were pushed down and internalized, but it was frustrated rage that lit the feelings on fire.

The body I live in now feels different. It is hard to describe how it feels to be here currently, except that in some ways it feels the opposite of before. I no longer turn the bulk of my aggression on my own skin. I am grounded in my feet more than most people, completely aware of my surroundings. Something is coiled and alive but relaxed within me, a sense that I can spring at a moment's notice if necessary, along with a sense that I won't have to, that I can't be sniffed out as a victim. I no longer carry that scent. The aggressive energy I have been able to harness throughout this journey has empowered me to stake a claim to myself, and to my right, my primitive need, to connect to others, and to love and be loved.

I hope that as you read, you will learn to care for those with BFRBDs from the roots up, to be mindful of the ways that attachment losses and pain may have detoured them from healthy development. If you can learn to sit with all the new and different and uncomfortable feelings you may have in the room with clients who pick, pull and bite, you can help them to move toward the development of new and healthier ways to relate to themselves and to others.

Moustakas (1990) explains how to assess the validity of heuristic research. This is done not through quantitative measures that can be determined by statistics but by a process of determining whether the depiction of the process to be validated is accurate, both to the researcher and to the constituents involved, in this case, the clients who participated in the case studies.

> The question of validity is one of meaning: Does the ultimate depiction of the experience derived from one's own rigorous, exhaustive self-searching and from the explications of others present comprehensively, vividly, and accurately the meanings and essences of the experience?
>
> (p. 32)

This book is the result of two decades of my heuristic research into the roots of BFRBDs. Part I focuses on understanding BFRBDs. Part II focuses on my treatment model, including applications in individual, family and group psychotherapy. My hope is that in this book I have accurately expressed my understanding of the meanings and essences of the struggle with BFRBs.

References

Bunker, J. (2021). Liberating ambition in women group psychotherapists. In Y. Kane, S. Masselink, & A. Weiss (Eds.), *Women, intersectionality and power in group therapy leadership* (pp. 123–138). New York, NY: Routledge.

Hill, C., Knox, K., & Pinto-Coelho, K. (2018). Therapist self-disclosure and intimacy: A qualitative meta-analysis. *Psychotherapy*, *55*(4), 445–460.

Morris, J. (2021). Cinderella, the wicked queen, and Glinda walk into a group: Countertransference resistance and the group leader. In Y. Kane, S. Masselink, & A. Weiss (Eds.), *Women, intersectionality and power in group therapy leadership* (pp. 108–122). New York, NY: Routledge.

Moustakas, C. (1990). *Heuristic research: Design, methodology, and applications*. Newbury Park, CA: Sage Publications, Inc.

Part 1

Understanding body-focused repetitive behavior disorders (BFRBDs)

1 The who, what, where, when, why and how of picking, pulling and biting behaviors

The 5 Ws and an H of body-focused repetitive behavior disorders

This year, when I was reading a new client's answers to an intake form, I noticed that she answered the question, "What do you want from therapy?" with, "I want to understand more about the 5 Ws and an H of my hair pulling." I couldn't figure out what she meant until we met, and she told me that she had been following my 2021 YouTube series and blog series, "The who, what, where, when, why, and how of body-focused behaviors," and liked my way of framing those questions. Some of these questions have clearer answers than others. In my heuristic journey to understand body-focused repetitive behavior disorders (BFRBDs), I was determined to find as many of these answers as possible. Presenting these questions and my understanding of the corresponding answers comprises the central aim of this book – to illuminate and guide therapists seeking to provide a depth-oriented approach to the treatment of these disorders.

1. Who (what population with what similarities) develops BFRBDs?
2. What are BFRBDs? Do experts have a common definition/diagnosis? What are the BFRB subtypes?
3. Where do BFRBDs occur (geographically; among which populations; under what conditions)? Where do people usually find themselves when their picking or pulling ritual begins (at home or at work)?
4. When (at what age) do BFRBDs tend to develop? What are common precipitating factors?
5. How do BFRBs substitute for more mature emotional regulation skills?
6. Why do BFRBDs develop?

The answers to those questions will differ depending on the theoretical approach one takes to the understanding of behavioral disorders. A

DOI: 10.4324/9781003299097-3

treatment model connects a theory about the etiology of a disorder with the goals of treatment, treatment methods and recommendations. In other words, a clinician's approach to treatment is grounded in her understanding of what causes a given disorder.

For some questions, about demography, common triggers for BFRBs and where they are likely to occur, I can answer with generally agreed-upon answers, drawn from the available literature. For other questions, like how to understand the BFRB automatic and focused subtypes, there is limited understanding and/or significant disagreement. In these cases, I answer the questions from my own perspective, and in the words of my clients. I also review how they have been answered from the cognitive-behavioral perspective, and, at times, from the developing field of psychodermatology. Though I have only recently become aware of the literature in this field, I have been amazed at the similarities between psychodermatologic assessments, definitions and treatment recommendations and my own.

My definition of body-focused repetitive behaviors comes from my grounding in the integrative psychodynamic approach I outline in Part 2 of this book. My theoretical perspective is attachment-based, relational and depth-oriented, thus leading to answers different from the ones that have been offered thus far through the traditional lens of cognitive-behavioral theory.

What are body-focused repetitive behaviors?

My definition: Body-focused repetitive behaviors are repetitive over-grooming acts, on the self-harm continuum, that serve as coping mechanisms. They do damage to the dermis. They are very effective in the short term in regulating physiological and emotional states and connect to a wide array of comorbid conditions. They include skin picking, hair pulling and cuticle/nail/cheek biting.

One element of this definition, that BFRBs are on the self-harm continuum, has proven controversial, as many in the BFRB field separate BFRBs from other self-harm behaviors like cutting. In my view, cutting is at one end of the continuum, where pain is a more conscious element of the desired result, with perhaps an unconscious motivation to cry for help, to express inner pain in an outward manner, and the experience of relief and release are side benefits. BFRBs tend to be at the other end of the continuum, with a focus on soothing, release and relief, and with the unconscious motivation to let frustrated energy out bit by bit. Pain is usually less of the desired result and more of an unintended effect. I specifically place both disorders on the same continuum to reduce the stigma of both poles of coping strategies involving bodily harm.

From the lens of an enhanced CBT approach, Jones et al. (2018) define trichotillomania and excoriation disorders as, "body-focused repetitive behavior (BFRB) disorders categorized by compulsive removal of hair and skin, respectively. Accompanied by either distress and/or functional impairment, these disorders are often quite burdensome to the individuals afflicted and are notoriously difficult to treat" (p. 728). This definition fails to capture many of the nuances in my definition, with a very clinical focus and divorced from the underlying psychological roots. The enhanced CBT lens is focused specifically on the behaviors themselves, while my lens focuses outward on how and why a relationship has been formed with behaviors that hurt the skin. The behavior-focused lens may well be why BFRBs have proven to be notoriously difficult to treat, because they are often related to complicated psychosocial factors that can't be fixed or solved in a few sessions.

My clients have had some insightful ways of defining their relationships with BFRBs. Em, who began pulling, chewing and eating their hair during a chaotic childhood says of their relationship with repetitive behaviors, "When I found hair pulling, I found a friend, a family, an acceptable soother. I never wanted to let it go." Em's description reflected the significance of hair pulling as a way to calm their central nervous system. Rose shared with me a metaphor for her hair pulling and skin picking behaviors calling them, her "blanket with thorns," emphasizing the comfort along with the pain. Both Em and Rose illuminated through these terms the power of their love-hate relationships with their body-focused behaviors.

While there are fundamental differences between my understanding of BFRBs and that of the researchers in the CBT field, we do agree that hair pulling and skin picking, along with cheek lip and nail-biting, would fit best in their own diagnostic category. Stein et al. (2010), some of whom are on the Scientific Advisory Board of TLC Foundation for BFRBs, advocated for the creation of a Body-Focused Repetitive Behaviors category in the *Diagnostic and Statistical Manual (DSM)* before the *DSM 5* was published (APA, 2013). BFRBDs have more in common with one another than with either their impulsive counterparts such as kleptomania or those under the obsessive-compulsive umbrella (OCD). They also are often found to co-occur (Roberts et al., 2013). Commonalities include physiological sensitivity and sensory processing disorder, as well as common comorbid conditions including depression, anxiety, body dysmorphic disorder (BDD), post-traumatic stress disorder, autism spectrum disorder and attention-deficit/ hyperactivity disorder (ADHD).

What are hair pulling, skin picking and nail/cheek/lip biting?

Picking, pulling and biting are normal human behaviors. This is because humans are, first and foremost, animals. Part of being an animal, whether an insect, reptile or mammal, is engaging in grooming behaviors, which serve a variety of functions including comfort, hygiene, self-expression and social connection (Natterson-Horowitz & Bowers, 2013). The behaviors only become problematic and reach clinical levels when they go beyond a grooming function and interfere with social or occupational development.

Physically, hair pulling is a sensory experience that involves pulling hair out of the scalp, lashes, brows or other areas with the fingers or tweezers. The behavior usually involves a pre-pulling ritual of searching for hairs with the desirable texture and characteristics, like gray, kinky or short. It is usually followed by a post-pulling ritual of manipulating the hair in some way, like running it through the fingers, pulling or biting off the hair bulb and feeling it, touching it to the lips or crunching it between the teeth, or chewing and swallowing the hair itself. Hair swallowing is also known as trichophagia and can create medical complications. The rituals and behaviors can involve all five senses: touch, taste, smell, sight and sound.

Skin picking is similar to hair pulling in both the pre- and post-picking rituals and engagement of multiple senses. It involves picking at acne, clogged pores, bumps, ingrown hairs, scabs or cuticles, with fingers, tweezers or other implements. Pre-picking rituals can include searching in the mirror for perceived imperfections or feeling for pickable spots. Post-picking rituals can include looking at, smelling and/or tasting sebum, scabs or blood, and picking too has potential medical consequences like infections that may need medical attention. Picking behaviors can also include nose-picking.

Cheek and lip biting, along with nail and cuticle biting, involve many sensations, from feeling or looking for an imperfection to chewing and swallowing nails or skin.

My descriptions of body-focused behaviors are explicit, and the visceral reactions you may have to the details are normal and instructive. In working with this client population, it is critical to face the discomfort head-on, forging a path for clients through shame and disgust. I have benefitted from talking out loud about this disgust, with colleagues and mentors, to shake off my own sense of it. For me personally, it is important to draw a boundary in sessions: we can talk about the ins and outs of BFRBs, but I request that people do not engage in the behaviors while we are together. That helps me to avoid feeling squeamish and helps to shift clients toward new possibilities of getting restless energy out of the body.

Many clients I have seen have kept the details of their behaviors, especially oral components, secret, for many years, within a wall of shame. To ameliorate this shame, when I meet with new clients, I list possible sensory elements in a matter-of-fact voice – an intervention that often helps them talk about the details of their own behaviors out loud for the first time and begins to break through the shame.

It is important, also, to be able to talk about the healthy grooming behaviors we also have in common with animals. In fact, healthy grooming is, perhaps, the most powerful antidote to unhealthy grooming behaviors. Natterson-Horowitz & Bowers explained, "In fact, human beings rely on this *release-relief* loop throughout the day. Stroking our hair, picking our toenails, chewing the inside of our cheek – these are powerful self-soothers" (p. 215). For humans, as with other animals, grooming provides a chemical bath for our nervous systems, literally relaxing us.

> Grooming actually alters the neurochemistry of our brains. It releases opiates into our bloodstreams. It decreases our blood pressure. It slows our breathing. Grooming someone else confers some of the same benefits. Even simply petting an animal has been found to relax people.
>
> (p. 214)

I will return to the animal–human connection throughout this book. As humans, we like to identify with our prefrontal cortex – that zone of wisdom and calculated decisions – rather than the brain stem that holds our animal instincts and impulses. Body-focused behaviors bring to mind images of monkeys picking fleas off one another, or a lizard shedding and consuming its skin.

Diagnosis

Defining BFRBDs diagnostically has been a challenging task for medical professionals, therapists and researchers, largely because they have both impulsive and compulsive features and overlap with so many other diagnoses. The first terms applied to hair pulling and skin picking, trichotillomania and dermatillomania, came from French dermatologists in the late 1800s. In a sign of how far behind the curve mental health treatment is, the first time a BFRBD appeared in the *DSM* was in the third revised version, under the category "impulse-control disorders (APA, 1987)."

McElroy et al. (1992) captured some of the similar features of the diagnoses in this grouping, including trichotillomania, as related to difficulty regulating affect, "The impulse control disorders not elsewhere classified appear to be related to one another and to mood, anxiety and psychoactive substance use disorders . . . . they may represent forms of affective spectrum disorder" (abstract). In the DSM's fifth edition, skin picking was finally included as "excoriation (skin picking) disorder," and both disorders were moved under the "obsessive-compulsive and related disorders" umbrella (APA, 2013).

Currently, for someone to receive one of these diagnoses, five conditions must be met. The following list is for the trichotillomania diagnosis:

1. Recurrent pulling out of one's hair, resulting in hair loss.
2. Repeated attempts to decrease or stop hair pulling.
3. The hair pulling causes clinically significant distress or impairment in social, occupational or other important areas of functioning.
4. The hair pulling or hair loss is not attributable to another medical condition.
5. The hair pulling is not better explained by symptoms of another mental disorder.

The criteria for excoriation (skin picking) disorder are very similar:

1. Recurrent skin picking, resulting in lesions.
2. Repeated attempts to decrease or stop skin picking.
3. The skin picking causes clinically significant distress or impairment in important areas of functioning.
4. The skin picking cannot be attributed to the physiologic effects of a substance or another medical condition.
5. The skin picking cannot be better explained by the symptoms of another mental disorder.

Also in 2013, the European Society for Dermatology and Psychiatry added a name and classification for the same skin-focused behavior. "Self-inflicted skin lesions (SISL)" are defined as "non-suicidal, conscious and direct damage to the skin" (Tomas-Aragones et al., 2017, p. 159). This society places the behavior along the self-harm continuum.

What are the BFRB subtypes?

Two subtypes of BFRBs have been identified, focused and automatic. They are distinguished by the impetus for the behavior as well as consciousness that it is happening. Focused BFRBs come from some conscious irritation with hair, skin and nails. The picking, pulling or biting focus is on remedying the perceived imperfection, whether in the mirror or by feel.

Automatic BFRBs are triggered unconsciously, as the first part of the ritual feel of skin or hair leads to a trance-like state in which time, perhaps hours, can be lost. A jolt back into reality leads to distress at the damage done. Either subtype can be more or less destructive to the dermis. Focus on a blemish with tweezers can do similar damage as spending hours pulling out hairs. Many people engage in both focused and automatic behaviors at different times.

There is general agreement that focused BFRBs have some overlap with OCD and BDD, in that they seem to have a role in shifting attention away from negative emotional states to focus on a blemish that has a short-term fix, that release/relief. This understanding has led to treatment recommendations to focus on building emotional regulation skills in an enhanced version of CBT (Jones et al., 2018).

Researchers have come to understand automatic BFRBs in two very different ways. Those from the CBT perspective have determined that automatic BFRBs are more like habits than responses to emotions. Thus, they hypothesize that behavioral treatments should be adequate to address automatic behaviors. As Jones et al. (2018) explain, "'automatic' pulling or picking behaviors being more habit-like and is engaged in with less conscious awareness . . . 'Focused' BFRBs are characterized as being engaged in more consciously and often serve to regulate uncomfortable physical sensations or emotions" (p. 729).

Separately, research from both the psychodermatology field and mental health field has been indicating a strong connection between the automatic subtype and PTSD, such that automatic behaviors are understood to be dissociative reactions to the intrusion of post-traumatic thoughts or feelings. As Özten et al. (2015) explain, the results of their study of around 60 people split among those diagnosed with skin picking, hair pulling and a control group, "We can conclude that trauma and PTSD may play a role in etiology of both TTM and SP . . . developing TTM or SP symptoms helps the patient to cope with intrusive thoughts related to trauma" (p. 1209).

Klosowska et al. (2021) added to this evidence,

> Our study provides support for the hypothesized relationship between trauma, dissociation and skin-picking behaviors in a non-clinical sample. We found that skin-picking is related to various types of traumatic events (emotional neglect, emotional abuse, bodily threat, sexual harassment), and that dissociative symptoms partly mediate this relationship.
>
> (conclusion)

This is a connection the Trichotillomania Learning Center (TLC) Foundation for BFRBs has resisted. Although trauma-focused cognitive-behavioral therapy is an evidence-based application of CBT, and although research connecting BFRBs and trauma has been building consistently since the early 2000s, the Scientific Advisory Board (SAB) has resisted acknowledging this connection. Eight authors including two members of the SAB published an article downplaying the connection, titled "Trauma and Trichotillomania: A tenuous relationship" (Houghton et al., 2016). Specifically, the articles challenged the connections drawn in my own case study (Nakell, 2015) and Oztën et al.'s (2015) findings. Their main conclusion was that rather than being linked directly to trauma, trauma leads to difficult emotions that in turn lead to BFRB engagement. From my perspective, that is exactly how PTSD symptoms develop, as a way to cope with the unbearable affect left behind by traumatic sequelae. The intent of the article seems to be to try to disconnect and distance these two intertwined elements of trauma.

Who/when/where

Researchers estimate that 0.6%–6.5% of the population struggle to some extent with BFRBs; the higher percentage includes manifestations of the behaviors that don't meet diagnostic criteria, such as those who pick or pull infrequently in ways that don't interfere with their lives (Roberts et al., 2013). Both disorders typically emerge in adolescence, though they can also emerge earlier in life – in children as young as 2 years old – or later in life. BFRBDs are four times more common in women than in men, though men may underreport, and some studies show a more equal gender distribution in trichotillomania (Grant et al., 2020).

Most research has focused on the prevalence and demographics of trichotillomania and skin picking separately.

In a study of more than 2,500 US adults 18 years and older, randomly selected, Keuthen et al. (2009) found that a high 11.2% of respondents endorsed at least one clinical skin picking event. This result warrants future research! It may be that this study captured the population who have engaged in some episodes of destructive skin picking without ever identifying the behavior as a mental health problem. It matches my own experience, in that many people who have sought me for therapy for other presenting issues also would have met the study's criteria for skin picking.

Grant et al. (2020) found that 1.7% of the general population of 18–69-year-olds met criteria for trichotillomania.

Studies in different countries, including Israel, China and Germany, indicate that BFRBDs are not confined to any specific culture (APA, 2013; Bohne et al., 2002). Comas-Díaz & Jacobsen (1991) note that a therapist's awareness of her own ethnocultural biases is a key element in treating all populations more effectively. The authors recommend that ethnicity, culture and race be considered directly as relevant variables in the consideration of any mental health diagnosis. A study of 41 African American women with trichotillomania found that in this population, anxiety and OCD symptoms were predictive of hair pulling severity (Neal-Barnett et al., 2011). The authors emphasize that cultural messages relating directly to the hair of the women impact their relationship with their hair. This and other studies indicate the need for future research on the ways BFRBDs can manifest in a range of communities and ethnicities.

There is limited information about a subset of children with early-onset trichotillomania. This group has been found to have different characteristics and comorbidities, thought to have more of a benign course, though recent research has indicated potential adolescent recurrences (Menon et al., 2015). More research into this subset is called for.

Most people begin to engage with problematic levels of picking, pulling or biting in early adolescence. We can presume that the rush of hormones has something to do with that, as emotions run high.

Women tend to notice fluctuations in BFRBs along with their menstrual cycles throughout life. During middle school and high school, acne is a common development, and pimples are there to be picked, easily becoming a focus of self-consciousness. At a time when belonging is a key developmental task, the sense of difference caused by obvious skin and hair damage increases social isolation. Preteens and teens may be less interested than their parents in working on their BFRBs and helping them to identify an internal motivation for change will be key to treatment.

Who will walk into your office?

I can only speak of those who walk into my office. I am a Caucasian female psychotherapist in Austin Texas, with less obvious identifiers Jewish, bisexual and gender fluid. My rates are similar to those of local therapists. When I was accepting new clients, I always offered sliding scale spots, most recently through the Open Path Collective. This is a national collective of therapists who offer at least one spot to people who couldn't otherwise afford therapy. Joining the collective brought much more diversity into my practice, in terms of age, race and socioeconomic status, and has been a gift. Around 70% of clients in my practice are Caucasian, and the other 30% are either mixed race, Black, or of Asian, Mexican, South American or Middle Eastern descent.

I work with preteens, teens and adults. The gender breakdown is roughly 80% female, 15% male and 5% somewhere on the non-binary gender continuum. Each has at least one comorbid condition, many have several versions of body-focused behavior, and the intensity of the behaviors when people enter treatment varies widely. Most of the adults who come to see me began to struggle with BFRBs as either preteens or teens, though several did experience pediatric symptoms and some developed BFRBs later in life.

Your clients struggling with BFRBs may have first tried to seek help from dermatologists for related medical issues. By the time they seek mental health treatment, they may have tried many prescribed medications and over-the-counter remedies to treat their skin. When depression and/or anxiety are also present, they may or may not have considered psychiatric treatment. Teens may have been lying to their parents about the cause of their hair loss and may have been diagnosed with alopecia before acknowledging their hair-pulling struggle.

Course and consequences

Engagement with BFRBs tends to bring short-term relief, and, over time, leads to negative long-term medical, social and emotional consequences. The medical consequences of hair pulling include bald spots on the scalp and eyelid infections, with rare but serious digestive issues resulting from hair consumption in cases of trichophagia. Skin picking can lead to difficulty in healing acne or wounds, infections and scarring. The emotional consequences include isolation, self-hatred, shame and secrecy.

BFRBs occur on a continuum, from minor – occasional pulling that isn't noticeable or that causes only superficial damage to the skin – to intense, which has major consequences. If hair pulling or skin picking are not accompanied by other stressors, they tend to be mild and not overly problematic. When accompanied by other psychosocial stressors, such as familial or academic stress, hair pulling and skin picking often worsen, abating only at times of relative calm (Roberts et al., 2013).

Without treatment, BFRB engagement often worsens throughout adolescence and adulthood. Bald spots or multiple scabs may be noticeable and become embarrassing. When the behaviors do begin in adolescence, physical markers such as bald spots or multiple scabs can become the focus of bullying and peer rejection. This dynamic leads to feelings of isolation at a time when the primary developmental goal is to achieve a sense of belonging.

Time spent on attempts to camouflage the damage to the dermis, whether extensive use of makeup or arrangement of hair or hairpieces, can intensify self-consciousness and limit participation in sports and water activities. Swimming or sweating can erase or disturb the carefully applied makeup or carefully arranged hair.

Many teenagers I work with find themselves bullied about their hair or skin. Some teens are so embarrassed by their appearance that they leave school and begin homeschooling, a decision that can add to their isolation and social anxiety.

Adults in the BFRB cycle may sometimes find their social struggles deepen, as they watch peers enter romantic relationships while they steer clear of intimacy for fear of revealing their secret behaviors. Thus, the consequences of BFRBs are often cyclical, difficult to change and are likely to worsen as stresses pile up and isolation deepens.

Why and how: emotional regulation model

The factors that lead to picking, pulling and biting involve some combination of nature (genetic) and nurture (environmental) factors. This combination is also known as diathesis/stress, as an underlying predisposition is brought out by an environmental stressor. The genetic underpinnings of BFRBDs are still being researched. Twin studies have shown a genetic link, and mutations found in the SLITRK1 gene have been linked to trichotillomania (Zuckner et al., 2006). Presumably, genetic mutations set the stage for BFRBs to erupt later in life.

In addition to these general issues, research has indicated some specific psychosocial stressors that tend to bring BFRBs out in force. Teens with trichotillomania describe having less freedom of emotional expression than their peers and also having stricter parents. The mothers of these teens tended to be more depressed and described greater than average family conflict (Keuthen et al., 2013).[1] Other experiences that contribute to the development of BFRBDs include trauma, the loss of a beloved attachment figure, divorce or a geographical move away from loved ones.

Grant et al. (2020) point to the high comorbidity rate as an important clinical consideration, "In general, the comorbidity data from this study are in keeping with previous studies showing that trichotillomania is frequently comorbid with multiple other mental health conditions, particularly OCD, anxiety, ADHD and PTSD" (p. 5). In their article organizing and reviewing the empirical research on the emotional regulation (ER) model for BFRBs, Roberts et al. (2013) comment on the extent of these comorbidities: "The results of studies exploring psychiatric comorbidity and psychological symptoms in individuals with BFRBs indicates that this population suffers from greater comorbidity and more psychological symptoms than are observed in control populations" (p. 758).

You will find that while BFRBs may be the presenting problem, they are usually only one piece of the psychological puzzle for these clients. It is likely that your client will present as accommodating and sweet, but once you scratch the surface, you will find that there are many untended feelings below. People who pick, pull and bite have learned, for one reason or another, that it is best to bottle up feelings that are deemed unacceptable, especially anger and frustration. So, rather than the behaviors serving as a cry for help, they tend to represent an effort to hide painful feelings. Picking, pulling and biting can all serve as ways to release tension and frustration bit by bit.

Those struggling with picking, pulling and biting share some other characteristics: difficulty with sensory processing from an early age, deficits in emotional regulation skills and personality traits of overachievement and perfectionism. Anger, specifically, is a difficult feeling for this population to regulate, whose tendency to direct anger toward the self is also the main trigger for BFRBs.

As we can see from the complicated emotional and relational experiences that precipitate BFRB engagement, picking, pulling and biting serve as coping mechanisms to manage a variety of stressors. Researchers have begun to coalesce around an emotional regulation (ER) model for BFRBs to explain how various stressors, including comorbid conditions, can combine to bring BFRBs out in force (Roberts et al., 2013).

This model matches what I have come to learn about BFRBs. They are remarkably effective at regulating physiological and emotional tension. The shift in feeling state can occur in any number of directions: ameliorating boredom by creating stimulation, returning to homeostasis after excitement or anxiety, zoning out to escape from intrusive thoughts or memories, focusing on a difficult problem or task, or releasing internal tension bit by bit. For any given person, BFRBs can serve any or all of these functions at different times, to manage different kinds of stressors.

In particular, anger seems to be a difficult emotion to regulate. In their study of 158 clinic-referred hair pullers between the ages of 18 and 65, Curley et al. (2016) found a significant correlation between difficulty expressing anger outwardly in healthy ways and severity of hair pulling.

In light of this study, the authors recommend that clinicians assess for deficits in ER and teach adaptive emotional regulation strategies in the treatment-planning process. They recommend CBT enhanced with acceptance and commitment therapy (ACT) and/or dialectical behavior therapy (DBT) for treatment. Psychodynamic treatment is grounded in attachment-based principals and, I will argue, is an even better fit to address some of the complex psychosocial dynamics that underlie difficulties with self-regulation.

Note

1. The authors noted that their research would have benefited from studying fathers as well as mothers. The focus on mothers reflects a bias that should be corrected in the future.

References

American Psychiatric Association. (1987). *Diagnostic and statistical manual of mental disorders* (3rd ed., text rev.). Arlington, VA: American Psychiatric Publishing.

American Psychiatric Association. (2013). *Diagnostic and statistical manual of mental disorders* (5th ed.). Arlington, VA: American Psychiatric Publishing.

Bohne, A., Wilhelm, S., Keuthen, N., Baer, L., & Jenike, M. (2002). Skin picking in German students: Prevalence, phenomenology, and associated characteristics. *Behavior Modification, 26*, 320–339.

Comas-Díaz, L., & Jacobsen, F. (1991). Ethnocultural transference and counter-transference in the therapeutic dyad. *American Journal of Orthopsychiatry, 61*(3), 392–402.

Curley, E., Tung, E., & Keuthen, N. (2016). Trait anger, anger expression, and anger control in trichotillomania: Evidence for the emotion regulation model. *Journal of Obsessive-Compulsive and Related Disorders, 9*, 77–81.

Grant, J., Dougherty, D., & Chamberlain, S. (2020). Prevalence, gender correlates, and co-morbidity of trichotillomania. *Psychiatry Research, 288*(112948). 10.1016/j.psychres.2020.112948.

Houghton, D., Mathew, A., Twohig, M., Saunders, S., Franklin, M., Compton, S., . . . & Woods, D. (2016). Trauma and trichotillomania: A tenuous relationship. *Journal of Obsessive-Compulsive and Related Disorders, 11*, 91–95.

Jones, G., Keuthen, N., & Greenberg, E. (2018). Assessment and treatment of trichotillomania (hair pulling disorder)and excoriation (skin picking disorder). *Clinics in Dermatology, 36*, 728–736.

Keuthen, N., Fama, J., Altenburger, E., Allen, A., Raff, A., & Pauls, D. (2013). Family environment in adolescent trichotillomania. *Journal of Obsessive-Compulsive and Related Disorders, 2*(4), 366–374.

Keuthen, N., Koran, L., Aboujaoude, E., Large, M., & Serpe, R. (2009) The prevalence of pathologic skin picking in US adults. *Comprehensive Psychiatry, 51*(2), 183–186.

Kłosowska, J., Antosz-Rekucka, R., Kałużna-Wielobób, A., & Prochwicz, K. (2021). Dissociative experiences mediate the relationship between traumatic life events and types of skin picking: Findings from non-clinical sample. *Frontiers in Psychiatry, 12*. https://doi.org/10.3389/fpsyt.2021.698543

McElroy, S., Hudson, J., Pope Jr., H., Keck Jr., P., & Aisley, H. (1992). The DSM-III-R impulse control disorders not elsewhere classified: Clinical characteristics and relation to other psychiatric disorders. *American Journal of Psychiatry, 149*(3), 318–327.

Menon, V., Shaik, S., & Mohan, P. (2015). Very early trichotillomania presenting with recurrent trichobezoar: Conventional wisdom questioned. *Journal of Trichology, 7*(1), 36–37.

Natterson-Horowitz, B., & Bowers, K. (2013). *Zoobiquity: The astonishing connection between human and animal health.* New York, NY: Vintage Books.

Neal-Barnett, A., Statom, D., & Stadulis, R. (2011). Trichotillomania symptoms in African American women: Are they related to anxiety and culture? *CNS Neuroscience & Therapeutics, 17*(4), 207–213. https://doi.org/10.1111/j.1755-5949.2010.00138.x

Özten, E., Sayar, G., Eryilmaz, G., Isik, S., & Karamustafalioglu, O. (2015). The relationship of psychological trauma with trichotillomania and skin picking. *Neuropsychiatric Disease and Treatment, 11*, 1203–1210.

Roberts, S., O'Connor, K., & Belanger, C. (2013). Emotion regulation and other psychological models for body-focused repetitive behaviors. *Clinical Psychology Review, 33*, 745–762.

Stein, D., Grant, J., Franklin, M., Keuthen, N., Lockner, C., Sincer, H., et al. (2010). Trichotillomania (hair-pulling disorder), skin picking disorder, and stereotypic movement disorder: Toward DSM-V. *Depression and Anxiety, 21*, 611–626.

Tomas-Aragones, L., Consoli, S. M., Console, S. G., Poot, F., Taube, K. M., . . . & Geiler, U. (2017). Self-inflicted lesions in dermatology: A management and thera-peutic approach : A position paper from the European Society for Dermatology and Psychiatry. *Acta Dermato-Venereologica.* DOI:10.2340/00015555–2522

Zuckner, S., Cuccaro, M., Tran-Viet, K., Cope, H., Krishnan, R., Parikac-Vance, M., et al. (2006). SLITRK1 mutations in trichotillomania. *Molecular Psychiatry, 11*, 888–889.

2   The psychic skin

Sensory processing, attachment and perfectionism in BFRBDs

Unanswered questions

Some important questions remain around the commonalities among people who struggle with BFRBs. Why, for example, do we so often see early difficulty with sensory processing coupled with later deficits in emotional regulation skills among this population? Why is anger a particularly difficult emotion for this population to regulate? And why is perfectionism such a common personality feature, with its hallmarks of "presenting a public face of cheerfulness, laughter, and a driven productivity?" (Hewitt et al., 2017, p. 235).

Sensory over-responsivity

Sensory processing difficulties seem to be key to the difficulties people with BFRBs experience with emotional regulation, but very few studies have examined this sensory element. Falkenstein et al. (2018) assessed the level of sensory over-responsivity (SOR) in a study of 1200 participants, half with trichotillomania and half in a control group. They defined SOR as, "a disproportionately intense, prolonged, or heightened reaction to ordinary sensory stimuli, such as tactile and auditory sensations" (p. 207). They found that the majority of those with trichotillomania experienced significantly higher auditory and tactile SOR than did those in the control group.

My clients describe different ways sensory processing difficulties manifested for them in childhood, often saying they hate the tags on the backs of clothing and the lining on socks. Sensitivity to food textures and to loud noises is not uncommon. People who engage in BFRBs often recall sucking on their thumbs or relying on a blankie for comfort as children, then struggling when these soothing mechanisms are no longer socially appropriate.

Elizabeth, who you will get to know in Chapter 6, traces her difficulty with self-regulation back to stories about her earliest experiences. She was

DOI: 10.4324/9781003299097-4

the fourth child born into a family with numerous stressors, with her own medical issues causing more stress,

> My parents were completely overwhelmed with job issues and money problems and children. So by the time I came along, and I was colicky, and I was described as a problematic baby, and I cried and I cried. And I had chronic ear infections, and I had surgery when I was one, and then I stopped crying so much. The way everyone talks about me as a baby, it was like, I just was a problem, I just couldn't get it together.

Attachment theory and emotional regulation

Falkenstein et al. (2018) note a connection between SOR, emotional regulation and perfectionism, while acknowledging that the links between the three are unclear. One hypothesis that rings true is that SOR symptoms lead to high levels of emotional arousal, which in turn leads to perfectionism as a maladaptive tool to regulate overwhelming emotions.

To better understand the connection between these dynamics, attachment theory is a good place to start. Attachment theory connects the ability to self-regulate emotions with the quality of early attachment relationships. According to this theory, "the attachment system evolved because it increased the likelihood that offspring would survive until they were old enough to reproduce and also taught children how to regulate emotions effectively" (Shaver & Mikulincer, 2014, p. 238). From this perspective, emotional regulation skills are developed in relationships with attachment figures from the very beginning of life.

Neurobiologists have affirmed this connection between early attachment relationships and the development of emotional regulation skills. As Schore (2003) explains, "Attachment is thus the dyadic (interactive) regulation of emotion" (p. 39).

My hypothesis is that early attachment disruptions, may well get in the way of this first stage of development for people who later develop BFRBDs. These disruptions can include unintended medical trauma, the disorienting loss of a grandparent, the loss itself compounded by taking its effect on a grieving parent, medical issues/hospitalization of the mother, postpartum depression, the difficult birth of a sibling, and/or unease or instability between the parents.

These types of disruptions at an early age can be unsettling to the central nervous system. Physiological sensitivity can lead to a number of other difficulties. The most sensitive person in the family often picks up on unexpressed feelings of other family members and may be the first to manifest signals that stress is high in the home. This person can easily become the identified patient or scapegoat of the family.

In addition, it is important to recognize that for someone with a sensitive central nervous system, adverse life events may well have a deeper impact. As a result, difficulty processing sensory stimulation can translate into difficulty regulating emotions. Early attachment disruptions can make it more difficult to be soothed throughout the more mature stages of emotional development. Because they often happen before words are available, they are unlikely to be named by clients as contributing factors.

As I weave these key threads together to enhance our understanding of the factors that may contribute to the development of BFRBDs, I want to be clear that I am not suggesting that these disruptions are a universal factor in the childhood experiences of those with BFRBDs. Rather, there are some intriguing clues within these connections, and my anecdotal experience leads me to suggest that the field would benefit from research into the early childhood experiences of those who later develop BFRBDs.

The psychic skin

Early attachment needs are largely met through the sensation of touch, through the medium of skin-to-skin contact with an attachment figure. The skin is full of nerve endings. Very receptive! It is also very vulnerable. The skin is literally the site of an infant's sense of the world. Esther Bick (1968), a modern analyst, wrote about the nuances of early attachment from her experiences treating infants. She was able to describe developmental processes that happen before a child can express those experiences in words. In particular, she gifted to the field her concept of the psychic skin.

The psychic skin is a critical first developmental step toward building emotional insulation. Imagine if, just as the skin grows along with the developing infant to serve as the first physical barrier to protect her from the world, there is also a psychic skin developing as a container to hold her developing self. Bick explains,

> The thesis is that in its most primitive form the parts of the personality are felt to have no binding force amongst themselves and must therefore be held together in a way that is experienced by them passively, by the skin functioning as a boundary.
>
> (p. 484)

There are two components to the development of a cohesive psychic skin. While the physical skin grows on its own, the psychic skin can grow only within a relational dance between the infant and the parent or attachment figure. For this to happen, the parent herself must be able to fully relax while holding the child. Feeding times are often when this kind of relaxation can occur, with the sensory elements of soothing in place: skin, smell, touch, taste and sounds. It is important to note that these sensory elements can all be met with or without breastfeeding. Bottle feeding, in cases where breastfeeding is not a viable option, can also incorporate all of the layers of sensation key to this sensory bath: touch, sound, skin-on-skin contact, the mirroring gaze and the movement of rocking.

In addition to providing a soothing space, an attachment figure must be able to help a child regulate painful feelings, whether she is screaming or inconsolable. This, in turn, means that parents must be able to tolerate both rage and despair in their children. As Schore (2003) explains, "the arousal-regulating primary caregiver must participate in interactive repair to regulate interactively induced stress states in the infant" (p. 39). This repair process helps to create a sense of containment, that even when strong feelings are experienced it will be okay, which in turn helps those feelings begin to subside. Thus, it is the capacity of the parent to provide a holding experience for the infant that in turn gives the infant access to deep relaxation, the seeds of the psychic skin.

Anzieu (1979) elucidates a similar idea of a skin ego, which serves two important functions: to hold the self together and to provide insulation from the outside world. Anzieu-Premmereur (2015) elaborates on this concept, explaining the deep connection between the development of the skin ego and the ability to regulate sensations and emotions. She describes the process, with "the skin-ego synthesizing stimuli and facilitating their regulation in order to contain states of over- or under-stimulation" (p. 672).

Welton and Kay (2015) elucidate the chemicals underlying this interplay,

> In humans, oxytocin is associated with a number of factors that affect attachment including trust, empathy, eye contact, and generosity. Oxytocin infusions in healthy individuals tend to decrease anxiety and the stress associated with social situations while shifting attention from negative to positive information.
>
> (First section, Paragraph 2)

In other words, we gain the ability to calm ourselves down through the experience of being calmed by a soothing other, and when we internalize this experience, our brains gain the ability to release the chemicals that bring about relaxation.

When I imagine the psychic skin, it's a soft, thick pink ribbon, transparent but cohesive, circling the infant completely. I imagine the emotional insulation that blooms from this first boundary as a more opaque, puttylike substance, growing wider and firmer throughout childhood development.

The aggressive drive and the narcissistic wound

Modern analytic theory may also offer a clue as to why anger and frustration might be such difficult emotions to regulate for those diagnosed with BFRBDs (Curley et al., 2016). In this model, one of the holes that can develop in the psychic skin is the frustration of the aggressive drive, leading to the internalization of aggression. The narcissistic wound is a name for this developmental block to assertion of the self (Spotnitz & Nagelberg, 1960).

Morris (2021) describes the development of the narcissistic wound,

> early emotional training leads to either stalled emotional development or healthy maturation, depending on the degree to which the child learns that frustration and anger can be directed safely outward without fear of destroying others or being destroyed by them. If we learn that such discharge is dangerous, a natural response is to turn the anger on oneself.
>
> (p. 114)

I visualize this compacted and internalized aggressive energy as a claw, embedded in one's chest like an ingrown toenail. I think of work with client aggression as helping to turn that claw outward, in the form of assertiveness, where anger as a signal can serve its natural function of self-protection.

Nagelberg & Spotnitz (1958) describe a therapeutic approach to helping clients discharge aggressive energy toward the therapist in order to release its grip on the self. "The psychic energy which has been so unprofitably invested in maintaining (stubborn infantile defenses against the release of aggressive impulses) can then be put at the ego's service for its own maturation and other desirable purposes" (p. 794).

This approach involves finding ways to engage with the client's preverbal self to restart the stymied process of discharge, such as joining, mirroring and connecting to nonverbal cues, all of which I incorporate into my integrative psychodynamic approach.

Secure and insecure attachment

For children of parents who can meet these early sensory and emotional needs in a nurturing environment, the early years provide a foundation for emotional regulation skills to grow and develop. Those who experience good-enough parenting develop a secure internal structure. These early relationship templates repeat later in life. Securely attached people have a sense of comfort in their own skin and a positive sense of self and expect and find mutual respect in their relationships.

Disruptions in this early development process are not uncommon. Parents can fail to create this preverbal holding space while trying their very hardest to be good parents. Bick (1968) noticed in her work with children that, no matter the parents' intentions, if this basic need wasn't fully met or was met but then disrupted by a loss or a family crisis, holes would develop in the psychic skin, hampering the ability of the baby to fully relax.

Karen (1998) outlined the results of an early experiment on children, Ainsworth's "the Strange Situation," to explain the outcome of secure and insecure attachment. The experiment involved the mother being with the child as a stranger enters the room, leaving the child with the stranger, and then returning to the room.

Although most of the babies explore the toys around them when their mothers are in the room, get closer to their moms when the stranger enters and cry when left alone with the stranger, those with secure attachments explore more freely than the others. The biggest difference in attachment style can be seen in how the child behaves when the mom returns to the room. The securely attached babies express their distress and can be calmed by their moms. The anxiously attached babies run to their moms, cling, and cry and cry, hard to soothe. The avoidant babies act like they don't see their moms and keep playing, but electrodes on their bodies show that they too are experiencing distress; they just hide it well. The babies with disorganized attachment structures have mixed reactions when their moms return, unsure of whether to approach or be afraid of her. Each of these attachment structures leads to defenses against intimacy. They just look very different.

Soft and hard comforts

Unlike those who develop secure attachments early on, those with insecure attachments struggle to self-soothe throughout life. In turn, they turn to compensatory strategies to calm their central nervous systems, finding hard comforts when soft ones are not available.

In Harry Harlow's famous monkey studies from the 1960s, he discovered that young monkeys preferred to be with a cloth stand-in mother than a wire one with a bottle. Although the cloth monkey couldn't attune to the babies like a real mother could, the experience of being held by another was possible, and these cloth mothers could meet a key developmental need (Karen, 1998).

The difference between Harlow's young monkeys' experiences with the wire monkey and the cloth monkey is that the cloth monkey was able to soothe and calm the baby. This is the very definition of a soft comfort.

In one of the Harlow's videos that is difficult to watch, a group of monkeys were allowed contact only with a wire monkey. They weren't very interested in the milk she had in a bottle. They screamed, endlessly, until the end of the video. In general, babies do tend to find replacement behaviors. If soft comforts are not available, they turn to hard comforts. Think of how babies need to wear mittens so they don't scratch themselves. Maybe when it takes a little too long to get a response from wailing, they begin to flail. Without mittens, there may be the discovery of some comfort in the pain of nails on skin, even an increase in endorphins, a feeling of release.

Flores (2004) established a connection between addiction and attachment disorders: "Certain individuals, because of intrapsychic or developmental deficiencies . . . are vulnerable to environmental influences (i.e., substance abuse), which further compromise an already fragile capacity for attachment" (p. 64). In this way, addictions can serve as hard comforts when soft comforts are not easily accessible.

Similarly, BFRBs can serve as hard comforts, helping to regulate emotions when soft, sweet ways of comforting have not been fully internalized. Anzieu-Premmereur (2015) describes a case in which trichotillomania serves to compensate for an insecure attachment, "For example, a fourteen-month-old baby was compulsively pulling his hair in a helpless search for self-soothing while experiencing the loss of his mother, who was emotionally unavailable" (p. 668). Promisingly, she described the reversal of this difficulty through treatment, "Therapy with baby and mother conjointly provided a framing background support in which this symptom disappeared" (p. 669).

Perfectionism and the false self

From my experience working with many clients who seem to have it all together, functioning at high levels academically and in social or professional organizations, with deeply unresolved feelings under the surface, I have come to understand perfectionism as a false self. Perfectionism is a way of hiding unacceptable feelings, including anger, behind a pleasing veneer. It is a way of coping that signals some sort of distress but, by its very nature, often falls under the radar. High-functioning students get positive attention, and this kind of behavior tends to be rewarded in society, unlike more obvious help-seeking behaviors such as using drugs.

For reasons we will continue to explore, those with BFRBDs have discovered that their relationships are more stable when they keep certain feelings, especially anger and frustration, tamped down. These feelings add to the inner tension boiling up inside, which makes it hard to tolerate strong emotions, and the outcome is social anxiety, isolation and a limited range of emotional expression.

Ester Bick (1968) provides a way to understand how perfectionism can stand in for healthier coping skills. Her idea is that damage to the psychic skin leads over time to the development of a false self, in which forced over-competence hides a less integrated state. Bick (1968) calls this false self a "second-skin formation" and described it as a hiding of dependency needs as compensatory behaviors develop. In this quote, "object" refers to a primary attachment figure,

> Disturbance in the primal skin-function can lead to a development to a 'second skin' formation in which dependence on the object is replaced by pseudo-independence, by the inappropriate use of certain mental functions, or perhaps innate talents, for the purpose of creating a substitute for this skin container function.
>
> (p. 484)

In these cases, compensations must be found to help a person get through life and tamp down unacceptable feelings. As we have learned, BFRBs can be very effective and adaptable compensations.

In their book *Perfectionism: A Relational Approach to Conceptualization, Assessment and Treatment*, Hewitt et al. (2017) further elucidate a psychodynamic understanding of perfectionism as a strategy to cope with early attachment disruptions. Although they don't address BFRBs specifically, they discuss how attachment disruptions in infancy can lead to perfectionism in adults.

The authors described the case of Amanda, who entered treatment for irritability and difficulty with social connections and was a serious overachiever. She had a sense that her mother was over-burdened at the beginning of her life, with her brother still a toddler, and remembered most of her childhood spent with nannies. No body-focused behaviors are listed in her case, but to me she sounds very familiar. The authors identified the roots of Amanda's drive for perfection in her early attachment experience,

> Amanda had lived her whole life acutely aware of a longing for her mother's love. The firm belief that her love for her mother was not reciprocated eroded Amanda's ability to embrace and find security in others' love for her. Her solution was to be perfect, while holding the simultaneous belief that others expected her to be perfect.
>
> (p. 245)

They described the success of Amanda's strategy of hiding her feelings behind a false, cheerful self in the short term, though it kept her from getting her emotional needs met in the long term, "As she got older, she discovered that putting herself at the service of others brought expressions of gratitude, while ensuring that no one was inconvenienced or burdened by her needs" (p. 248).

The authors pointed to a strong therapeutic alliance, helping clients see both the positives and negatives of perfectionism in order to move past the perfectionism defense toward a deeper layer of feeling as key to treatment success. "What are often not expressed overtly are feelings of anger, fear, sadness, or even disgust . . . With patients like Amanda, we make the assumption that there are deeper and more intense emotions beneath what is first expressed" (pp. 235–236).

Before we turn to the integrative psychodynamic approach, it will be helpful to review the history of treatment until this point, through the dermatology, psychiatry and mental health fields.

References

Anzieu, D. (1979). *The skin-ego.* New York, NY: Routledge.
Anzieu-Premmereur, C. (2015). The skin-ego: Dyadic sensuality, trauma in infancy, and adult narcissistic issues. *Psychoanalytic Review, 102*(5), 659–681.
Bick, E. (1968). The experience of the skin in early object-relations. *International Journal of Psychoanalysis, 49,* 484–486.
Curley, E., Tung, E., & Keuthen, N. (2016). Trait anger, anger expression, and anger control in trichotillomania: Evidence for the emotion regulation model. *Journal of Obsessive-Compulsive and Related Disorders, 9,* 77–81.
Falkenstein, M., Conelea, C., Garner, L., & Haaga, D. (2018). Sensory over-responsivity in trichotillomania (hair-pulling disorder). *Psychiatry Research, 260,* 207–218.
Flores, P. (2004). *Addiction as an attachment disorder.* Lanham, MD: Jason Aronson.
Hewitt, P., Flett, G., & Mikail, S. (2017). *Perfectionism: A relational approach to conceptualization, assessment and treatment.* New York, NY: The Guilford Press.
Karen, R. (1998). *Becoming attached: First relationships and how they shape our capacity to love.* New York, NY: Oxford University Press.
Morris, J. (2021). Cinderella, the wicked queen, and Glinda walk into a group: Countertransference resistance and the group leader. In Y. Kane, S. Masselink, & A. Weiss (Eds.), *Women, intersectionality and power in group therapy leadership* (pp. 108–122). New York, NY: Routledge.
Nagelberg, L., & Spotnitz, H. (1958). Strengthening the ego through the release of frustration-aggression. *American Journal of Orthopsychiatry, 28*(4), 794–801.
Schore, A. (2003). *Affect regulation and the repair of the self.* New York, NY: W. W. Norton & Company.
Shaver, P., & Mikulincer, M. (2014). Adult attachment and emotion regulation. In J. J. Gross (Ed.), *Handbook of emotion regulation* (pp. 237–250). New York, NY: The Guilford Press.
Spotnitz, H., & Nagelberg, L. (1960). A preanalytic technique for resolving the narcissistic defense. *Psychiatry: Interpersonal and Biological Processes, 23*(2), 193–197.
Welton, R., & Kay, J. (2015). The neurobiology of psychotherapy. *Psychiatric Times, 32*(10), at www.psychiatrictimes.com/view/neurobiology-psychotherapy

3   The history of BFRBD treatment

Dermatological treatment

In addition to being the ones to name the disorders trichotillomania and dermatillomania, dermatologists were the first to treat them. Still to this day, many people first seek treatment for the symptoms of BFRBs, the bald spots or infections, from medical professionals without even knowing there is a mental health component of the disorders.

Beginning in the 1880s, BFRBs were being diagnosed and treated not as psychological conditions but as physical injuries. People struggling with BFRBs would seek help either at doctors or, even more commonly, at dermatologists' offices for help. Traditionally, dermatology has fallen under the medical model where illnesses are to be remedied or "fixed." Damage from skin picking and hair pulling was treated with topical or oral medications, along with the message to the patient to stop picking or pulling. Dermatologists initially attempted to treat the disorders in this way for some time but found that that approach did very little to reduce hair-pulling and skin-picking behaviors (Orion et al., 2012).

Almost a century later, in the 1960s, psychiatrists also began to attempt to solve the trichotillomania puzzle. Pharmacological treatments have been studied for decades, with little success. Anti-depressants and anti-anxiety medications have, to some extent, helped reduce comorbid conditions, but they have not proven successful in reducing picking or pulling behaviors themselves (Stemberger et al., 2003).

In the mid-twentieth century, both dermatologists and psychiatrists began to recognize that the psychosocial and mental health factors contributing to BFRBDs went beyond what they – or their science – were equipped to handle. In medical terms, dermatologists recognized the "influence of psychosocial stress in the exacerbation or chronicity of skin illness" (Rodríguez-Cerdeira et al., 2011, p. 22), but they could not pinpoint the precise connection. Psychiatrists had learned that stress could trigger physical disorders such as

DOI: 10.4324/9781003299097-5

psoriasis, and, conversely, dermatological symptoms could create emotional distress, which in turn could exacerbate symptoms.

These complexities led to the creation of a new medical field: psychodermatology. A psychodermatology approach includes psychiatric and psychological care along with medical treatment. Psychodermatologists treat their patients holistically, with a focus on support and understanding, as well as shame reduction, while also addressing the skin issues at hand. Orion et al. (2012) explain: "A psychodermatology clinic is the format that enables dermatology patients to receive a comprehensive approach to their skin condition as well as to the difficulties it imposes on their lives, and vice versa" (p. 97). In other words, psychodermatology works to address the complex psychosocial factors that factor into the development of BFRBDs.

Mental health treatment

On the psychological side, in the 1970s, clinicians began to focus on how to treat trichotillomania, though it would be another decade before hair pulling was included in the *DSM* (APA, 1987), and even longer for skin picking (APA, 2013.) At that time, therapists from the two major schools of psychological thought, psychoanalysis and behaviorism, were beginning to treat hair pulling (not skin picking yet). Each approach had markedly different answers to etiology, assessment, goals and interventions with this population.

In the 1970s, Freudian psychoanalysis was the primary form of treatment for any number of disorders. Freudian analysis served as the basis for "talk therapy" and provided a foundation for modern psychodynamic work. Freudian analysts understand disordered behaviors as symptoms of deeper issues, deriving from unconscious drives and unresolved psychosexual problems. Freud saw self-destructive behaviors as an outgrowth of anger turned inward due to an early relational failure, with aggressive energy that was unacceptable to parents turned back on the self (Nagelberg & Spotnitz, 1958).

When psychoanalysts began to treat people with trichotillomania, they made several important contributions to our evolving understanding of the disorder. For one, they postulated that the etiology of hair pulling stemmed from disruptions in primary relationships. This hypothesis fit with the main precipitants for BFRBDs that often included the loss of loved ones, divorce or illness in the family, or the loss of social support (Jafferany & Osuagwu, 2017).

Psychoanalytic assessment focused on identifying the comorbid conditions common among those with BFRBs and attending to the stressors at play when the behavior developed, including attachment losses and family crises. The goal of therapy was to uncover the unconscious roots of the hair-pulling behavior to release the grip of the behavior on the psyche. Interventions involved encouraging a free flow of associations between hair pulling and any symbolism that could explain its emotional meaning to the patient, to explore the connections between these dynamics and the self-destructive behaviors.

Psychoanalysis provided an explanation for the difficulty of letting go of body-focused behaviors. Problematic behaviors were understood to be coping mechanisms that were difficult to part with. Resistance to change arises hand in hand with the possibility of change, and if a therapist tries to tackle dysfunctional behaviors before clients are ready, resistance will become entrenched.

However, there were several serious problems with psychoanalytic treatment at that time. The Freudian focus on underlying psychosexual conflicts, such as penis envy and fear of castration, was too narrow to account for the various triggers for BFRBs. Talk therapy at the time was focused solely on words without grounding in the body and failed to address the dysregulated nervous system endemic in this population. Traditionally, analytic conversations about the roots of behaviors might lead to an insight into the connection to early psychosocial conflicts, but the insights themselves didn't lead to behavioral change (Keuthen et al., 1999).

At the same time, around the 1970s, behaviorism was developing as an alternative to psychoanalysis for treating a number of behavioral disorders. Behaviorism was in many ways a polar-opposite approach. It was designed to address the problematic behaviors themselves, without concern for their underlying roots.

In contrast to the psychoanalytic focus on symbolism and the unconscious, behaviorism was grounded in the work of B. F. Skinner, who attributed the etiology of disordered behaviors to experiences of sensory reward and punishment resulting from them. In short, if a behavior creates a positive feeling, it will likely continue. If it is paired with a negative experience, for example, a small shock, it will be extinguished.

Behavioral assessment focused on identifying the intensity and triggers for problematic behaviors, and the primary goal was the elimination of these behaviors. Interventions involved punishment for the behaviors and rewards for engagement in healthier alternative behaviors. Therapeutic interventions were manualized and oriented toward finding behavioral solutions to hair pulling, with a focus on worksheets and homework to track the frequency of behaviors over time and to implement replacement strategies.

Since the creation of the Trichotillomania Learning Center (now the TLC Foundation for BFRBs) in 1990 and its Scientific Advisory Board soon thereafter, resources have been directed toward research and treatment grounded in the behavioral approach. This approach is based on an understanding of BFRBs as the issue at hand, rather than as symptoms of deeper psychological or psychosocial issues.

At that point, the psychoanalytic approach was left behind. The TLC Foundation has consistently advocated for the use of cognitive-behavioral therapy (CBT) with this population, excluding psychodynamic treatment as an evidence-based option.[1]

In the mid-1990s, Dr. Nathan Azrin, a preeminent behaviorist, expanded his application of techniques based on operant conditioning, stimulus response and reinforcement specifically for the treatment of trichotillomania in a version of behavioral therapy known as habit reversal therapy (HRT)/stimulus control (SC) (Peterson et al., 1994).

The habit reversal approach had one goal: the extinction of body-focused behaviors. Keuthen et al. (1999) clarified this perspective: "Behavioral therapists have focused exclusively on the target behavior without hypothesizing masked unconscious conflicts. The hair pulling itself has been defined as the problem rather than as a symptom of a more fundamental conflict" (p. 148).

The HRT/SC technique incorporated four main interventions toward this goal: awareness training, competing response training, social support and stimulus control interventions (Snorrason et al., 2015). Briefly, these involved noticing the immediate antecedents to pulling, performing an action – such as clenching the fists – that is incompatible with pulling when the antecedent occurs, bringing a support person in to help with awareness and eliminating triggers in the environment.

HRT brought in some important treatment components: awareness training and the need for social support. In the 1980s, when HRT/SC became the gold standard for treatment for this population, studies measuring the amount and intensity of hair pulling in an 8- to 16-week protocol showed positive results. Typically, about 30% of those who reduced or extinguished the behaviors were able to maintain their improvement, particularly those whose symptom intensity was at the mild end of the continuum or who stopped hair pulling completely by the end of the program.

However, longer-term studies revealed that these gains were often reversed, as relapses were common after the first 3 to 6 months post-treatment (Mansueto et al., 1999). For 50%–70% of patients, relapse and/or the development of a cross-addiction (such as overeating and abusing alcohol) complicated the treatment picture (Roberts et al., 2013).

Trying for bettter results, Charles Mansueto, founder and director of the Behavioral Therapy Center of Greater Washington, took the lead in developing a comprehensive protocol for addressing some of the commonalities between people who pick and pull. He added to HRT the cognitive, sensory and emotional components of BFRBDs. He called this protocol ComB, for comprehensive behavioral therapy (Mansueto et al., 1999).

The comprehensive behavioral program, ComB, is a protocol in which the therapist assesses five categories that contribute to BFRBDs: motor, environment, affect, cognitive and sensory. With the therapist, clients identify triggers for their picking or pulling behaviors in each of these categories. Once triggers are identified, clients list ways to distract from, cope with or change the triggering elements, either in session or for homework. The job of the therapist is to then help brainstorm and find solutions in each of these categories. As Keuthen et al. (1999) explained, "Attention is focused on the situational and emotional triggers for the disorder and on the mechanisms of reinforcement by which the behavior is maintained" (p. 148).

For example, if hair pulling occurs when someone is feeling sad or lonely, therapist recommendations might include calling a friend or engaging in an enjoyable activity. Sensory elements, such as stress balls and other fidget toys, are incorporated into the intervention toolbox. Cognitive interventions bring attention to thought patterns that sustain picking or pulling episodes, such as "I'll just pull this one hair," or "I've already pulled my hair and ruined my progress, I may as well keep going."

Again, applying the ComB protocol looked promising, but progress wasn't maintained over time (Roberts et al., 2013). It became clear that some of the triggers listed on the ComB worksheet were complex psychosocial stressors that couldn't be resolved within the worksheet format, and that extinguishing problematic behaviors would not be as easy as initially hoped.

Limitations of the CBT approach

Though emotions were included in the ComB protocol, the model focused on a limited range of emotional regulation skills, mostly related to shifting away from negative feeling states. In their literature review, Roberts et al. (2013) explained that a limited goal of emotional regulation can be counterproductive: "The distinction between ER as emotional control/suppression and ER as awareness and understanding is critical because some literature suggests that efforts to control emotional experience and efforts to avoid or reject uncomfortable emotions may underlie psychological symptoms" (pp. 749–750).

Also, as discussed in Chapter 1, there has been a resistance in the behavioral field to acknowledging the intimate connection between trauma and BFRBs, and a trauma-informed approach has been lacking. "The basic difference between a trauma-informed approach and the traditional perspective . . . is that the traumatic event or experience is never viewed as irrelevant to understanding and treating behavioral or mental health problems," Courtois and Ford (2013) explain in their seminal work *Treatment of Complex Trauma: A Sequenced, Relationship-Based Approach*.

This means that people who experience BFRBs may be anywhere on the continuum, from never having experienced trauma, to having gone through something awful but recovering without trauma symptoms, to being diagnosed with PTSD as a primary diagnosis, to experiencing chronic attachment shock. Özten et al. (2015) describe the connection between automatic picking and pulling and the dissociative effects of trauma, making the case that trauma should be considered a significant precipitating factor for BFRBDs. I never assume a traumatic history; instead, I assess for and treat traumatic symptoms rather than letting them fall through the cracks.

Ultimately, in many cases, the focus on behavioral change had the unintended side effect of creating more shame about the behaviors. It is difficult to capture in words the devastation of growing out one's eyelashes for months only to pull them all out in a pulling relapse binge. These sorts of highs and lows can be incredibly discouraging and embarrassing and will certainly interfere with the treatment process. It became clear to many clinicians and researchers that self-compassion must be included in the mix, and those body-focused behaviors needed to be understood as coping strategies rather than problems to be eradicated.

As a result, newer evidenced-based practices, including DBT and ACT, have now been integrated into ComB treatment programs. Both additions expand the viewpoint from the singular goal of symptom reduction to attending to the whole person in their psychosocial environment. Enhanced versions of ComB have shown promise in both reducing behaviors and maintaining reduced engagement in the behaviors.

Bottesi et al. (2020) performed a single-case experimental design study with three participants with trichotillomania. They utilized an 8-week ComB protocol and added in relapse prevention techniques as well as specific interventions to reduce shame, build self-compassion and manage stress. Of the three, one, whose hair pulling was manageable at baseline, benefitted from internalizing positive self-talk. The other two experienced ups and downs with pulling based on the stressors they faced during and post-treatment and gained more tools to cope with these stressors.

Keuthen et al. (2010) described the results of ten female subjects with trichotillomania who went through a DBT-enhanced CBT program. The program had 11 weekly individual sessions and 3 follow-up sessions. They found that this combination led to significant and sustained improvement in both hair pulling and emotional regulation overall, with treatment gains sustained throughout maintenance for 3 months post-treatment, with some mixed results 6 months post-treatment.

I am heartened to see that these enhanced approaches are more successful at reducing BFRB symptoms and reducing the unfortunate success/

relapse cycle. For people whose struggles with BFRBs are not entangled with attachment disruptions or trauma, an enhanced ComB approach may well meet their needs and lead to lasting resolution of BFRB symptoms.

However, these treatments are still focused on body-focused repetitive behaviors as the problems to be solved rather than as symptoms of underlying psychic wounds. From a psychodynamic perspective, this separation of the symptoms from their roots is a mistake, as the exploration of the roots of behavioral symptoms is the very pathway to healing on a deeper level. Although attachment disruptions are a frequent precipitating factor for BFRB development, the enhanced behavioral approach does not prioritize the therapeutic relationship as a healing factor.

Adaptive emotional regulation

Roberts et al. (2013) suggest that a more comprehensive idea of emotional regulation – adaptive emotional regulation – may be better suited to the complex emotional dysregulation faced by pickers and pullers. They explain that through this wider lens, "ER is defined by the ability to experience, differentiate between, and respond spontaneously to the full range of emotional experiences . . . Adaptive ER may therefore require acceptance of both pleasant and unpleasant responses" (pp. 749–750).

Adaptive regulation skills are based on mindfulness and tolerance of a wide range of emotions and take into account the psychosocial context of a given situation. Roberts et al. (2013) explain, "Adaptive ER therefore requires context-dependent flexibility, and strategic modulation of arousal in order to maintain goal-directed activity and inhibit impulsive behavior when negative emotions develop" (p. 750).

These complex relational skills are those my integrative psychodynamic approach addresses within the healing power of the therapeutic alliance. The therapeutic alliance has been consistently shown to be a predicator of therapeutic success (Safran & Muran, 2000). Jafferany & Osuagwu (2020) suggested that psychodynamic therapy may be a good fit for working with BFRBs because the model, "focuses on childhood experiences, personal fantasies, and unconscious conflicts. These underlying feelings play a major role in many psychiatric conditions including TTM and other obsessive-compulsive related disorders" (p. 4). And so, on to a new approach!

Note

1. The TLC Foundation Scientific Advisory Board's "Expert Consensus Treatment Guidelines: Body Focused-Repetitive Behaviors: Hair Pulling, Skin Picking, and Related Disorders" can be found at www.bfrb.org/storage/documents/Expert_Consensus_Treatment_Guidelines_2016w.pdf

References

American Psychiatric Association. (1987). *Diagnostic and statistical manual of mental disorders* (3rd ed., text rev.). Arlington, VA: American Psychiatric Publishing.

American Psychiatric Association. (2013). *Diagnostic and statistical manual of mental disorders* (5th ed.). Arlington, VA: American Psychiatric Publishing.

Bottesi, G., Ouimet, A., Cerea, S., Granziol, U., Carraro, E., Sica, C., & Shisi, M. (2020). Comprehensive behavioral therapy of trichotillomania: A multiple-baseline single-case experimental design. *Frontiers in Psychology, 11*. https://doi.org/10.3389/fpsyg.2020.01210

Courtois, C., & Ford, J. (2013). *Treatment of complex trauma: A sequenced, relationship-based approach.* New York, NY: Guilford Press.

Jafferany, M., Mkhoyan, R., Stamu-O'Brian, C., & Carniciu, S. (2020). Nonpharmacological treatment approach in trichotillomania (hair-pulling disorder). *Dermatologic Therapy.* https://doi.org/10.1111/dth.13622

Jafferany, M., & Osuagwu, F. (2017). Trichotillomania: Basic concepts. In K. Franca & M. Jafferany (Eds.), *Trichotillomania (hair pulling disorder)* (pp. 17–34). Hauppauge, NY: Nova Science Publishers.

Keuthen, N., Aronowitz, B., Badenock, J., & Wilhelm, S. (1999). Behavioral treatment for trichotillomania. In D. Stein, G. Christenson, & E. Hollander (Eds.), *Trichotillomania* (pp. 147–166). Washington, DC: American Psychiatric Press.

Keuthen, N., Rothbaum, B., Falkenstein, M., Meunier, S., Timpano, K., Jenike, M., & Shaw Welch, S. (2010). DBT-enhanced habit reversal treatment for trichotillomania: 3- and 6-month follow-up results. *Depression and Anxiety, 0*, 1–4.

Mansueto, C., Golumb, R. G., McCombs, A., Townsley Stemberger, T., & Townsley Stemberger, M. (1999). A comprehensive model for behavioral treatment of trichotillomania. *Cognitive and Behavioral Practice, 6*, 23–43.

Nagelberg, L., & Spotnitz, H. (1958). Strengthening the ego through the release of frustration-aggression. *American Journal of Orthopsychiatry, 28*(4), 794–801.

Orion, E., Feldman, B., Ronni, W., & Orrit, B. A. (2012). A psychodermatology clinic: The concept, the format, and our observations from Israel. *American Journal of Clinical Dermatology, 13*(2), 97–101.

Özten, E., Sayar, G., Eryilmaz, G., Isik, S., & Karamustafalioglu, O. (2015). The relationship of psychological trauma with trichotillomania and skin picking. *Neuropsychiatric Disease and Treatment, 11*, 1203–1210.

Peterson, A., Campise, R., & Azrin, N. (1994) Behavioral and pharmacological treatments for tic and habit disorders: A review. *Developmental and Behavioral Pediatrics, 15*(6), 430–441.

Roberts, S., O'Connor, K., & Belanger, C. (2013). Emotion regulation and other psychological models for body-focused repetitive behaviors. *Clinical Psychology Review, 33*, 745–762.

Rodríguez-Cerdeira, C., Pera-Grasa, J. T., Molares, A., Isa-Isa, R., & Arenas-Guzmán, R. (2011). Psychodermatology: Past, present and future. *Open Dermatology Journal, 5*, 21–27.

Safran, J., & Muran, J. (2000). *Negotiating the therapeutic alliance: A relational treatment guide.* New York, NY: Guilford Press.

Snorrason, I., Berlin, G., & Lee, H. (2015). Optimizing psychological interventions for trichotillomania (hair-pulling disorder): An update on current empirical status. *Psychology Research and Behavior Management*, *8*, 105–113.

Stemberger, R., Stein, D., & Mansueto, C. (2003). Behavioral and pharmacological treatment for trichotillomania. *Brief Treatment and Crisis Intervention*, *3*, 339–352.

Part 2

Integrative psychodynamic treatment for BFRBDs

4 Integrative psychodynamic therapy

A relational path to earned secure attachment

Psychodynamic theory is complex. The word itself includes a reference to psychoanalysis, which indicates the primacy of the therapeutic relationship and the exploration of the unconscious. In the modern version of psychodynamic therapy, the therapist's role goes beyond the "blank slate" therapeutic stance of psychoanalysis and into a more mutual engagement. Therapist joins and validates the client in the development of goals and encourages conversations about feelings and projections that arise in the relationship.

The term "psychodynamic" comes from the idea of thermodynamics, which refers to heat as a force of movement and transformation of materials. Psychodynamic therapy similarly embodies the principle that forces, motives and energy generated by the deepest of human needs contribute to disordered behaviors and mental states (Klimek, 1979).

Because it is hard to measure less tangible results like one's quality of life and relationships, psychodynamic theory isn't backed by as much evidence as CBT. The research that exists, however, does show that a slower, relational change process can lead to long-term positive results, by self-report, with many populations. Psychodynamic treatment has proven effective for many conditions, including somatic disorders, complex mental disorders, depression, anxiety, eating disorders and even personality disorders (Shedler, 2010).

Therapeutic gains in these areas tend to be sustained when assessed 5 years post-treatment. Shedler describes this success: "The evidence indicates that the benefits of psychodynamic treatment are lasting and not transitory and appear to extend beyond symptom remission. For many people, psychodynamic therapy may foster inner resources and capacities that allow richer, freer, and more fulfilling lives" (p. 107).

In practice, psychodynamic treatment is flexible rather than dogmatic. The theory has been shaped by the recent evolution of attachment theory, neurobiological research, somatic theory and trauma research. Psychodynamic

DOI: 10.4324/9781003299097-7

therapy is not manualized; instead, the therapist provides a container in which therapeutic work unfolds. Because it is individualized, this approach is eclectic and uses, tools from a variety of treatment modalities, including cognitive and behavioral therapies.

Psychodynamic treatment is continuously evolving, integrating new techniques and deepening the clinical understanding of the workings of the human psyche. In this way, it's an ideal model that allows us to embrace clients where they are and offer them a blend of various approaches to suit their needs.

Trauma and BFRBs

From a trauma-informed perspective, there are clear connections between BFRBs and trauma, as PTSD is a common comorbid condition. As Courtois and Ford (2013) make clear, "The basic difference between a trauma-informed approach and the traditional perspective . . . is that the traumatic event or experience is never viewed as irrelevant to understanding and treating behavioral or mental health problems" (p. 55).

This means that people who experience BFRBs may be anywhere on the continuum, from never having experienced trauma, to having gone through something awful but recovering without trauma symptoms, to being diagnosed with PTSD as a primary diagnosis, to experiencing chronic attachment shock. Özten et al. (2015) make the case that trauma should be considered a significant precipitating factor for BFRBDs. I never assume a traumatic history; instead, I assess for and treat traumatic symptoms rather than letting them fall through the cracks.

Evidence for the psychodynamic approach

In the position paper of the European Society for Dermatology and Psychiatry, Tomas-Aragones et al. (2017) establish the benefits of utilizing a psychodynamic approach for complex cases of BFRBDs. "If there are life-long problems, specific problems with emotional communication, or if underlying anxieties appear, patients with acne excoriée, trichotillomania or another disorder belonging to the compulsive spectrum of [self-inflicted skin lesions] SISL might benefit from psychodynamic therapy" (p. 166).

The psychodynamic treatment approach to BFRBDs has rarely been studied, perhaps because the results are not as easily measured as when the goal is symptom elimination, and researchers often dismiss it altogether. I am one of the very few people who have written about the benefits of this approach. Researchers in the field of psychodermatology have been including my approach in their treatment recommendations, and more data on this topic are sure to be forthcoming.

Those who did come before me saw very positive treatment outcomes in small studies. Caroline Koblenzer relied on case studies to reflect on the important benefits of psychodynamic treatment in her chapter in the book *Trichotillomania* (1999), making a strong argument:

> I have previously reported a positive outcome in four patients out of a series of six similar patients who accepted referral for psychodynamic psychotherapy . . . These therapies have repeatedly been demonstrated to be effective in the treatment of trichotillomania.
>
> (p. 142)

In a more recently published case study, Saya et al. (2018) set forth the positive results of psychodynamic treatment with a 45-year-old woman who had been pulling her hair since the age of 12:

> Her feelings of desperation and anguish, and the rather dramatic expression of them, accompanied by constant suicidal ideas, reveal other conflicts in her primary relationships. The contact with these relational issues is accompanied by a progressive resolution of the trichotillomania. This also comes through in the significantly symbolic shift from the pulling of her own hair to the pulling of the hair from her wig.
>
> (p. 214)

This case reflects the depth and symbology of psychodynamic work – the clinician followed the patient's symptoms as guideposts to understanding her relational needs.

I co-authored a write-up of the case study of Colt, featured in Chapter 8 (Aukerman et al. 2021). The conclusion was that psychodynamic therapy should be considered an evidenced-based treatment option,

> Combined approaches are popular, and this case report serves as evidence that a primarily therapeutic approach has the potential to be highly effective. It is important to approach trichotillomania multidimensionally and ensure that patients are referred to psychiatric services if they present to dermatology clinics.
>
> (last paragraph)

The "talking cure" and affective and somatic awareness

Psychodynamic treatment has been known as the "talking cure" because of its clinical focus on putting feelings and thoughts into words. This form of honest, spontaneous conversation plays a significant role in my work, as it does in all psychotherapy. Narrative therapy is the modality that is woven throughout our conversations. In asking my clients to share their thoughts and feelings about current and past events, I get to know the stories behind critical moments in their social and emotional development. As we go along, I also learn how they relied on picking or pulling to help them through those moments.

In addition to verbal communication, however, my approach corrects some of the flaws in traditional psychoanalysis by grounding treatment in somatic and affective awareness. Monk and Zamani (2019) explain that an updated version of narrative therapy includes an "affective turn" in which mind, body and emotions are all included in the storytelling New stories emerge in the process. For example, they point out that in order to process the kind of fear response that occurs in difficult or traumatic experiences we must locate the memory of fear in the body. I think of this as an embodied narrative process.

Zimmerman (2018) cites literature that shows the effectiveness of this embodied narrative approach, "Productive narrative processing of emotion predicts the best outcomes; experiencing emotions and then building narratives around them contribute to the best results" (p. 54).

In my office, the process of embodiment includes several elements: helping clients with body awareness during sessions, bringing body language into the conversation and being aware of my own body, both as a guide to what the client may be feeling and as a regulator. For example, as I work to help my clients breathe deeply and to be with their feelings instead of disengaging from them, I breathe with them. My calm body can help regulate their body. Words alone will not always suffice.

This process of talking along with somatic awareness helps clients connect the dots between their triggers and their behaviors. Two examples will bring you into the room with me. When 12-year-old Caucasian female Sarah came in with a new bald spot, I asked what led her to pull her hair more than usual. She cried as she told me her parents had realized she was allergic to her pet bunny, and she had to say goodbye to the bunny when it went to another home.

New possibilities for coping came to light after she told the story, as she showed me a series of memes she had found on her phone about cute bunnies talking with their owners. She imagined out loud a meme about letting her bunny know how much she loves her, and we laughed together.

Lesley, a mixed-race woman in her thirties who had been seeing me for over a year, was embarrassed to tell me a secret she had kept about her habit as an adolescent of keeping scabs from her own wounds in a little box. She was disgusted by her behavior and wondered if I would think of her as a freak. Instead, I asked what was going on in her life at the time this habit formed. She cried as she talked about how her mother's boyfriend had moved into their small house and how she consistently felt like a bother when she needed attention. She had buried her pain in that little box, and she experienced great relief when we revisited and processed those memories.

As was the case with Sarah and Lesley, deeper expression of affect often includes physical release of pent-up emotions, such as crying, yelling or laughing. My role in the room is to be a safe person to witness and experience painful feelings with. It is important to remember that feelings that feel intolerable alone can be detoxified and made tolerable within, and only within, a relationship.

An integrative psychodynamic approach

Sharon Ziv-Beiman (2015) was the first to introduce integrative psychotherapy as a particularly useful model in working with body-focused repetitive behaviors in a case study featuring Dana, a 23 year old woman with resistant trichotillomania.

In her model, the theories and treatment interventions Ziv-Beiman weaves together include strategic, cognitive, behavioral, dialectical and psychodynamic elements. Treatment is grounded in the therapeutic relationship, a foundation on which adaptive emotional skills can blossom.

She explains her grounding in cyclical psychodynamics theory. "In a mutual interaction, present experiences and relational configurations impact the psychodynamic infrastructure, the latter concurrently shaping the person's behavior, experiences in the real world, and interpersonal relationships" (p. 180).

This complex theory explains how the therapeutic alliance can serve as a foundation for corrective emotional experiences, as reflected in the case study, "The new patterns of interaction that Dana and I developed facilitated the therapeutic change. In contrast to her internalized authority figure, I was an authoritative female" (p. 180).

While there are many short-term goals to explore along the way, the long-term goal of integrative psychodynamic therapy is to fill in gaps in development, toward an earned secure attachment.

This process happens through transference and countertransference in the therapeutic relationship. The term transference describes the way clients project their experiences with early attachment figures onto the therapist, creating space for the transformation of these experiences. For example, if a client's father's reaction to her expression of angry feelings was to shut down, she will expect the same from the therapist. This will come out in avoidance of conflict in the therapeutic relationship. I make clear from the first session that I am sure to say or do something that will annoy or frustrate each of my clients, and that I want to know when that happens. This early invitation opens the pathway for more honest communication between us than is familiar.

Countertransference refers to the therapist's internal responses to her clients, which can run the gamut of uncomfortable feelings, including love, frustration, disgust, attraction and hopelessness. The ability to hold and sort through these feelings is a critical therapeutic skill, one that helps us to understand both the suppressed feelings of the client's body (congruent countertransference) and the feelings that significant attachment figures may have had toward them (concordant countertransference). These feelings are then available for us to process and release. As we repair therapeutic ruptures, old scripts can be rewritten, leading to new ways of relating to others.

As I tend to the transference and countertransference dynamics with clients with body-focused repetitive behaviors, I find that nonverbal expressions and physical sensations in my own body provide important clues. Joining each person's experience is an important therapeutic tool, helping clients to access early, even preverbal, experiences (Ormont, 2001).

Andi, who will also be featured in Chapter 9, came to see me when she was 26. She was in distress about pulling and eating her hair since the age of 10. After relying for so long on hair pulling as a way of coping, Andi had little access to her emotions. In particular, she viewed anger and sadness as negative feelings to be avoided. She was a very pleasant and hardworking person and tried to stay on the surface as she talked about her life. I joined her in this tentative pace, asking object-oriented questions about her life (What did you say? How did that go for you?) rather than talking too much about emotions.

The first glimmer of Andi's deeper emotions became noticeable in the ways that her words didn't line up with her body language, as she would share a difficult experience and then laugh, while also tearing up. Sometimes, I would feel my own throat close as Andi talked about her relationship with her mother.

When I gently mentioned these physical sensations within sessions, Andi was able to get in touch with the rage and grief she had experienced as a sensitive child growing up with a controlling and critical mother and absent father.

Eventually, we came to understand Andi's act of pulling out and eating her hair as a way of coping with the intensity of her anger, which had been unwelcome in her family environment. My accepting and inviting stance led her to try expressing her anger toward me more directly. In time, she talked about ways she was asserting herself more in her relationships. In turn, this shift led to reduced urges to pull her hair, even when she was angry.

Resistance and relapse

One element we are sure to encounter with our clients is resistance. Resistance is the desire to cling to unhealthy behaviors and choose the status quo over change. Resistance is a factor even if that change is ultimately what they want – to get better, to have better skin, to grow their hair back.

Behaviorists working with this population tend to view the ongoing pattern of success during treatment followed by relapses as a failure on the client's part to comply with the skills learned in therapy. Relapse work involves the reengagement with these strategies (Woods & Twohig, 2008). In my experience, there is an important step missing. Paying attention to resistance throughout treatment is one of the best ways to avoid relapse!

The concept of resistance is one of Freud's enduring contributions to the field. Freud recognized that we all have defenses to keep us protected from feelings and experiences that might make us too vulnerable or that are too scary to face directly. He also understood that if these defenses are challenged head-on, resistance will emerge in force. The best way to deal with resistance is to join it.

Resistance with pickers, pullers and biters tends to manifest as over-compliance. When perfectionists enter a program with behavioral goals, they tend to follow through on their desire to please by over-compliance with the therapist. Thus, it is key to go slowly, shift from a goal-oriented perspective, explore all the ways picking or pulling has been helpful, and set realistic expectations that picking and pulling will not immediately get better.

In her case formulation of Dana, who had experienced some success in reducing symptoms after working with a CBT therapist, only to suffer a devastating relapse, Ziv-Beitman decided to bypass the symptom as a target of treatment. She explained this as a way to respect the importance of hair pulling as a coping mechanism and also sidestep resistance,

> I suggest that sometimes, bypassing the symptom may allow processes of change that had previously been arrested . . . In such cases, focusing on the symptoms may unwillingly strengthen the pathological equilibrium, the therapy itself thus contributing to the problem.
>
> (p. 175)

I join my clients' hatred of their behaviors and their desire to get rid of them, how difficult they have made life, while adding a compassionate lens about their role as coping mechanism. In this way, I can stay out of the tug-of-war of trying to take soothing behaviors away. I offer behavioral and sensory tools from the first session but leave it to each client to pick them up to find what might work for them when they are ready.

It is difficult to capture in words the devastation of growing out one's eyelashes for months only to pull them all out in a pulling relapse binge. These sorts of highs and lows can be incredibly discouraging and embarrassing and will certainly interfere with the treatment process. When we respect our clients' resistance, we can avoid dragging them into the trap of failed attempts to get rid of unwanted behaviors. Down the road, as I continue to find ways to join clients' resistance to changing behaviors, they begin to turn toward that change on their own.

Three phases of treatment

A safety phase is a key element of any trauma-informed treatment approach. I need to make sure my clients and I have a positive alliance before focusing on behavioral symptoms or stepping into trauma work. As a therapist, one of my primary duties to my clients is to do no harm. Trying to eliminate a behavior before understanding the role it serves can be harmful. It is not uncommon for a teen or adult client to find me after feeling like they had failed at cognitive-behavioral therapy with a previous therapist. I attribute much of these chronic negative outcomes to the lack of a safety phase.

This stage has components that are key to building trust, whether trauma is in the picture or not. During the first few weeks or months, we work through shame and introduce self-compassion. We lay the groundwork for healthier coping mechanisms. This phase allows time for a comprehensive assessment, realistic goal formation, and the establishment of trust and connection between us.

The safety phase can be minimal if trauma is not involved, or it can be extended, depending on the intensity of trauma symptoms. We will explore the safety phase more fully in Chapter 5.

The second phase, the exploration and intervention phase, makes up the bulk of treatment. This phase can include a variety of treatment modalities, such as art, family and group, and is the focus of Chapters 6–8. Adaptive emotional regulation strategies such as expression and modulation are built and strengthened in this stage. Relationship skills are put into practice both in the therapy room and in clients' lives.

As I work to understand each person's unique patterns of picking and pulling, I encourage them to express all their thoughts, feelings and associations. As a result, they begin to release some of the tension in their bodies and move through unprocessed feelings. Many find at this point that it becomes more natural to try on healthier soothing behaviors, including positive grooming activities such as massages, warm baths and hair care. My slower approach helps me sidestep resistance, as clients try out new behaviors independently, through their own curiosity, rather than me assigning them.

In this phase, we also attend to communication and assertiveness skills and work toward modulation of responses to stressful situations. We move more deeply into resolution of trauma and complicated grief.

The third phase of treatment is the adjournment phase, which leads to either ending the therapeutic work or continuing in maintenance treatment. We will explore this phase in Chapter 9.

Hope for change

Neurobiologists have discovered that the brain retains plasticity later in life, and that new attachments can lead to literal changes in the brain, which in turn set the template for healthier relationships. As Flores (2004) explains, "If affect-regulation and self-soothing are internalized, the person will be less dependent on external sources for gratification" (p. 67). So, we can help our clients internalize our care, which in turn will help them to find and accept healthier versions of grooming and self-soothing behaviors.

A number of clients have told me they begin to think "What would Stacy say?" when assessing their response to a situation. My positive regard for them and my acceptance of their feelings open new options for my clients to assert themselves.

This is the beauty of all the hard work of being present in our own bodies in the room with our clients. If we can find a way to be with them that increases their internal sense of security, they can change their internal scripts and get more of what they want in life. A psychodynamic therapist supports healing on a level deeper than picking and pulling. In turn, this takes the pressure off the urges to pick and pull.

References

Aukerman, E., Nakell, S., & Jafferany, M. (2021). Psychodynamic approach in the treatment of trichotillomania. *Dermatologic Therapy*. DOI:10.1111/dth.15218

Courtois, C., & Ford, J. (2013). *Treatment of complex trauma: A sequenced, relationship-based approach*. New York, NY: Guilford Press.

Flores, P. (2004). *Addiction as an attachment disorder*. Lanham, MD: Jason Aronson, Inc.

Klimek, D. (1979). *Beneath mate selection and marriage: Unconscious motives in human pairing*. New York, NY: Van Nostrand Reinhold.

Koblenzer, C. (1999). Psychoanalytic perspectives on trichotillomania. In D. Stein, G. Christenson, & E. Hollander (Eds.), *Trichotillomania* (pp. 125–146). Washington, DC: American Psychiatric Press, Inc.

Monk, G., & Zamani, N. (2019) Narrative therapy and the affective turn: Part 1. *Journal of Systemic Therapies*, *38*(2), 1–19.

Ormont, L. R. (2001). *The technique of group treatment: The collected papers of Louis R. Ormont, Ph.D.* Furgerim, L. (Ed.). Madison, CT: Psychosocial Press.

Özten, E., Sayar, G., Eryilmaz, G., Isik, S., & Karamustafalioglu, O. (2015). The relationship of psychological trauma with trichotillomania and skin picking. *Neuropsychiatric Disease and Treatment*, *11*, 1203–1210.

Saya, A., Siracusano, A., Niolu, C., & Ribolsi, M. (2018). The psychodynamic significance of trichotillomania: A case study. *Rivista di Psichiatria, 53*, 214–217.

Shedler, J. (2010). The efficacy of psychodynamic psychotherapy. *American Psychologist, 65*(2), 98–109.

Tomas-Aragones, L., Consoli, S. M., Consoli, S. G., Poot, F., Taube, L., Linder, D., . . . & Gieler, U. (2017). Self-inflicted lesions in dermatology: A management and therapeutic approach: A position paper from the European Society for Dermatology and Psychiatry. *Acta Dermato-Venereologica, 97*, 159–172.

Woods, D., & Twohig, M. (2008). *Trichotillomania: An ACT-enhanced behavior therapy approach therapist guide (treatments that work)*. New York, NY: Oxford University Press.

Zimmerman, J. (2018). *Neuro-narrative therapy: New possibilities for emotion-filled conversations*. New York, NY: WW Norton & Co.

Ziv-Beiman, S. (2015). Integrative psychotherapy and coping with pathological syndromes: Dilemmas around the treatment of a patient with resistant trichotillomania. *Journal of Psychotherapy Integration, 25*(3), 175–182.

5 The safety phase
Goal-setting, assessment and self-compassion

Setting the stage

My relationship with each client begins even before we meet in person or on a video call, whenever they reach out to see if I am the right therapist for them. My first question when we do meet is always, "How did you feel about coming here to see me today?"

I have found that setting the stage for the end of treatment during the very first session can greatly reduce the likelihood that therapy will end without a goodbye. As we go over the counseling agreement, I mention to my clients that sometimes they won't want to come to see me, and that when they feel that way, I'd like them to come and tell me about why they didn't want to come.

This gives us a chance to understand how therapy is going – perhaps they are feeling overwhelmed, and we need to change our pacing, or maybe I said something that irritated them and we need to talk about it. This process has the added benefit of welcoming them to express negative feelings toward me when they arise, which allows them to process emotions they usually don't allow anyone to see.

When we talk about the course of therapy, I clarify that treatment length varies, and that 6 months to 1 year of weekly sessions is the minimum for a successful course of treatment. I ask them to let me know when they start to feel they are done with our work so that we can talk it through together. I also mention that I always like to have a closure session to honor our work together and say goodbye.

My first clinical interventions are mostly related to mirroring and joining, modern analytic concepts that help us start the process at the first emotional level of the psychic skin. My job at this phase is to helping clients feel seen and heard as we begin to get to know one another. Flores (2004) describes this relational process, "If there is an authentic, genuine attachment relationship, the patient's behavior and attachment style should trigger in the

DOI: 10.4324/9781003299097-8

therapist a genuine emotional response that matches the 'tune' the patient is playing" (p. 157).

The therapeutic alliance is built on a foundation of a safe attachment relationship between therapist and client and strengthened through agreement on goals and tasks of therapy (Summers & Barber 2003). From start to finish, the quality of our therapeutic alliance remains a priority in my mind. In this first phase, we are setting the foundation for repairing relational wounds, restoring, in a sense, the psychic skin. I help my clients create a safer buffer between the self and the world. Together, we work on meeting the most primitive of needs: to experience full-body relaxation, to be comforted when distressed and to have even the most painful and ugly of emotions accepted and understood.

Setting goals

Goals for therapy are addressed in the first one or two sessions. While I validate the urgent need to get rid of body-focused behaviors, I am honest about the need to set moderate behavioral goals. I think about the best outcome in terms of reducing reliance on picking and pulling behaviors and building more adaptive ways to cope. I also mention that when new stressors arise, we are always more likely to fall back into body-focused behaviors.

Goal-focused work that tracks behaviors can feed the perfectionism that is part of the problem; on the other hand, the idea of accepting some level of picking or pulling while reducing intensity and negative consequences can lead to a healthier new direction.

I like to view success in moderate terms: reducing the urges to pick and pull and building more skills to deal with stressful situations and painful emotions. Urges to pick and pull tend to fluctuate along with life's stressors. I explain that our first order of business will not be to focus on the behavior at all, because first we have to shake off some shame and learn self-compassion when picking or pulling is impossible to resist.

Eventually, my clients and I come to an agreement on these attainable goals. We examine how picking or pulling has helped them to regulate their nervous systems and manage difficult emotions such as anger and sorrow. Body-focused repetitive behaviors are so compelling because they actually do provide comfort in the short term.

Instead of the idea of getting rid of a behavior, I explain that we will do better if we focus on healthier replacements for that behavior. This starts with finding other things to do with our restless hands, and gradually becoming more aware of feelings, learning to tolerate our wide range of emotions, expressing feelings in productive ways, asserting needs in relationships, and modulating and sublimating emotions.

Throughout the three phases, I draw on different types of interventions. The tools for the safety phase include meeting immediate sensory needs, including with fiddle toys, working on basic co-regulation through breath work and psychoeducation.

In this phase, I am working on a number of tasks with my client: collaborating to create goals, taking a full assessment, creating a psychodynamic case formulation and helping the client shift from shame to self-compassion.

Full assessment

A full assessment takes into account the many layers of each individual's experience. It begins with the questions on my assessment forms and continues in my observations and conversations with them.

Some therapists administer assessment tools before, during and after the treatment process. I prefer to go through my assessment in conversations throughout the process. The assessment tools that may be most useful in psychodynamic work are the Difficulties in Emotional Regulation Scale and the Self-Compassion Scale – Short Form, both of which can be purchased through NovoPsych. Other helpful assessment tools include the Adult Attachment Interview (Main, 1991) and Motivational Interviewing (Miller & Rollnick, 2013).

Jones et al. (2018) expanded their recommendation for enhanced cognitive-behavioral therapy (CBT) to include more than a behavioral assessment. They recommend that in addition to assessing the frequency, intensity and consequences of the BFRBs and related medical issues or skin conditions, a clinical interview should include attention to past treatment experiences, medications and comorbid conditions. They note the importance of understanding both the automatic and focused subtypes. They frame automatic BFRBs as habit-like and more easily resolved through behavioral interventions rather than as PTSD symptoms; however, they do not include trauma screening as part of the recommended assessment. They also mention that clinicians should be aware of the high levels of shame that tend to be connected to BFRBs and to be sensitive in the assessment process, "Embarrassment and shame in these disorders are common, and so taking extra care in the interview will facilitate greater self-disclosure" (p. 729).

Psychodynamic case formulation

A psychodynamic case formulation goes deeper than the CBT assessment. Summers (2018) describes the three crucial parts of a case formulation, all of which I include in my assessment questions. Part 1 includes a summary of the current problem in the context of the client's life and development, including "identifying information, events precipitating the illness, extent and quality of interpersonal relationships, and predisposing factors" (p. 44). Part 2 focuses on the non-dynamic factors that may contribute to the problem and includes an understanding of the client's temperament, history of psychiatric and medical illness in the family, and history of trauma. Part 3 captures the central conflicts in the person's life, developmental difficulties and main psychological defenses. The author emphasizes that recent research indicates that these parts of understanding each person's core issues all overlap. Thus, early temperamental and neurobiological issues will impact how each person copes with the ongoing stressors of life. For example, "Childhood OCD may intensify separation difficulties because of a profound need for reassurance and alternatively a sense of premature autonomy and aloneness" (p. 45).

The assessment allows us to develop a sense of the relational and attachment framework a client brings to the treatment. By starting at the roots of the problem and building our way to the behavior, we bypass resistance and facilitate the therapeutic alliance. Summers (2018) explains,

> the updated formulation will increase the modern patient's awareness of the role of both psychological and neurobiologic factors in his or her life and experience and would be a first pass at glimpsing the complex understanding that might be gained in a successful treatment.
>
> (p. 50)

Ziv-Beiman (2015) lets the reader into her psychodynamic case formulation of client Dana who we met in Chapter 4. You will note the complexities of the picture she describes,

> The psychodynamic formulation I constructed was based on the special role assigned to Dana in the family. Her birth was a kind of miracle for her parents. Her mother had been traumatized first by her abandonment as a child and then again by the alienation and loneliness she experienced on the kibbutz.
>
> (p. 177)

Ziv-Beiman also described the way she understood this background to factor into the development of trichotillomania symptoms, "The TTM also symbolizes Dana's own aggression and sexual drives-expressed in the satisfaction it gives her" (p. 177). I would agree that sexual drives can be a factor, though not universally, in some cases. In any case, I too seek to understand the roots of the frustrated aggressive energy that comes out of restless hands.

Areas to assess/questions/follow-ups

Thus, a full assessment considers the many layers of each individual's experience. It begins with the questions on my assessment forms and continues in my observations and conversations with them. Each therapist must find her own rhythm and clinical voice for gathering the information to create the case formulation and treatment plan.

Our initial conversations tend to paint a picture of the daily stressors that trigger each person's picking, pulling or biting behaviors. These stressors might include school or work, primary relationships, commutes and computer time along with other disruptions. I want to understand how picking or pulling helps each person cope with these stressors.

At some point, I will want to know details about the picking or pulling ritual. This will help me understand the sensory and emotional needs being met before, during and after picking or pulling episodes.

The following are some areas I typically assess, along with some suggestions for questions to get more information and areas that may need follow-up referrals.

Behavioral

Questions: How often do you pull your hair? Do you focus for a few minutes or hours? Do you sometimes feel like you go into a trance? What parts of the sensory experience do you get pleasure and/or relief from? How much distress do you feel about hair pulling? How much does it get in the way of your life?

Follow-ups: Referral to physician? Dermatologist?

Sensory elements

Comorbidity

Questions: Current anxiety and depression symptoms? Self-esteem? Issues with food? Other substances? Sensory processing issues?

Follow-ups: Referral to a local psychiatrist/psychiatric nurse practitioner? Nutritionist?

Past experiences with therapy

Genetic factors

Questions: Other family members with BFRBs and/or comorbid conditions?

Interpersonal relationships

Temperament

Questions: Relationship status? Friendships? Current relationship with members of family of origin? Living situation?

Current triggers

Questions: When and where do you usually find yourself pulling out your hair? What do you notice happens in your body, or emotionally, before you pull? What are you thinking about during the episodes?

Defenses against difficult feelings

Intersections of marginalized identities

Questions: What are your current and previous experiences with gender, sexual orientation and racial discrimination? How do you experience your own hair and skin?

Precipitating factors

Attachment style

Questions: What were your experiences with your family of origin? How were your first 2 years of development?

Shame level

Questions: Who in your life knows about your hair pulling? How have those people responded? Have you gotten unwelcome attention about your hair?

Trauma

Because trauma assessment is not a typical element of the assessment of BFRBs and yet is critical to include, a deeper dive into the process is called for. Dissociation in sessions is a cue that PTSD is in the mix. If clients are dissociative (glazed eyes, long pauses, no eye contact), I first work on grounding, very basic body awareness, taking deep breaths and having them look at me while we breathe. It would be counterproductive to let them talk about their traumatic memories at this point. This early on, I would gently stop a new client from launching into the specific stories that weigh heaviest on their psyches.

I emphasize that we will return to these important stories, but that first they need to get to know me, we need to build trust, and we need to go slowly. This intervention is usually well received. In order to heal from trauma and to get its residue out of the body, they need to connect their trauma narrative with their emotions, be in their body and feel connected to me while it is happening.

Research shows that this is the only way to release traumatic residue from the body and fully resolve post-traumatic symptoms. As Courtois and Ford (2013) explain, "Emotion processing enables the client to safely experience and appraise in present time the physical sensations, emotions and thoughts that he or she had interpreted as signals of overwhelming danger and associated powerlessness" (p. 151). This process happens only after safety in the therapeutic alliance has been established.

Case example

The complexity of the ongoing assessment process and case formulation is best captured through a case example. Let's look at the information I gathered during the first two sessions with my client Maria.

Maria, an amalgamation of several clients, is a 27-year-old second-generation Mexican American female. In our first session, Maria presented as very cheerful and sweet, which didn't seem congruent with the history of major depressive episodes she described. She had suicidal ideations in the past but not since starting anti-depressants during college.

She wore a baseball cap to our first session. She seemed nervous as she started talking about her hair pulling. She told me that the pulling from her scalp was out of control. She began to notice bald spots, had to start wearing a cap to hide them and decided to seek help. She giggled awkwardly as she talked about the bald spots. The pulling had gotten worse this year, after she uprooted herself from her hometown and moved to Austin, where she now had a stressful job and few social connections. She moved away from home partly to explore her identity as bisexual, as she didn't feel comfortable including her parents in that part of her life.

When I asked if there were any exceptions to her experience of loneliness in Austin, Maria brightened and talked about finding a jazz band to play with. She told me she had always loved playing the saxophone and had played it throughout high school and college. She had been trying to date but hadn't made any romantic connections since her move.

Maria explained that her last experience in therapy didn't end well. She had tried CBT to help with her hair pulling and was very motivated to keep track of her behaviors. She stopped pulling out her hair, and her therapist told her happily that she had met her goals and was done with therapy. She didn't feel done but she didn't tell the therapist that. She began pulling her hair again on her car ride home.

In our second session, Maria told me what she remembered about the experiences that preceded her hair pulling. She described her childhood in terms of before and after her parents' divorce when she was 12. Before, she had been happy, with a minor habit of biting her nails that wasn't a big problem. After, she developed a binge-eating disorder, and at the age of 13 developed bulimia. At 16 she entered a treatment program. She was diagnosed with depression, began taking anti-depressants and was able to develop a healthier relationship with food. It was at that point that her body-focused behavior shifted from nail-biting to hair pulling.

My case formulation for Maria begins to form. The loss Maria experienced when her "happy family" dissolved hasn't been processed emotionally; rather, she turned to body-focused and other behaviors to cope with the pain. She has discovered that people-pleasing and perfectionism are effective defenses against less comfortable feelings like anger. She has a great deal of shame about her hair pulling, and it has led to a cycle of self-hatred and isolation. She has many strengths and had a foundation of stability before the divorce that engendered resilience. Acceptance of her sexual orientation has been difficult, as in her Catholic upbringing homosexuality was defined as a sin and bisexuality was never mentioned.

Therapeutic plan

In an integrative approach, the psychodynamic case formulation informs the therapeutic plan moving forward. What we learn about clients' attachment structures, the precipitating factors that led to the BFRB, and the psychosocial and sociocultural factors that impact them in this phase, we apply in the skill-building phase of treatment. Ziv-Beiman (2015) frames the process of integrating the formulation and plan beautifully in her case study of Dana, the 23-year-old female with severe trichotillomania we met in Chapter 4,

> Taking into account . . . the psychodynamic formulation of Dana's world . . . my evaluation that Dana possesses solid and effective ego strengths . . . and the immediate positive bond that I experienced in my early relationship with her . . . I chose to devise a treatment that combined strategic intervention, interpretative work around the psychodynamic formulation, cognitive challenging, augmenting her self-esteem . . . and corrective experiences.
>
> (p. 178)

The therapeutic plan for Maria would include many of these same interventions. I would add an additional early focus on building beginning emotional regulation skills like awareness and tolerance of difficult feelings and replacing shame with self-compassion, along with a later stage focus on working through trauma and helping her to build assertiveness and conflict resolution skills.

First task: co-regulation

I encourage co-regulation of the nervous system through simple breath work and body awareness for all my clients, not only those who come in with acute trauma symptoms. Giving clients tools to begin to sit with and be aware of their feelings through co-regulation sets the stage for the development of emotional regulation.

The relationship is the "magic treasure chest" (as Anna, featured in Chapters 6 and 9, named it) full of helping tools we may discover in any given session. This includes attention to transference and countertransference. Ruptures in our relationship (some version of the client getting mad at me and us talking it out) are ongoing, as is my interest in the current stressors in their lives. Through this dynamic process, we are replacing the shame about picking, pulling or biting with self-compassion.

Replacing shame with self-compassion

Shame is the experience of thinking that we are bad. Shame expert Brené Brown (2007) explained, "Shame is the intensely painful feeling or experience of believing we are flawed and therefore unworthy of acceptance and belonging" (p. 27). Shame is sticky and gets in the way of letting go of body-focused behaviors.

Shame is a negative internal experience that can trigger picking or pulling and picking and pulling in turn create more shame. I am often the first person a client has risked confiding in about their behaviors. Sometimes they have revealed themselves to someone whose reaction added another layer of shame.

Luckily, there is an antidote to shame: self-compassion. Kristin Neff (2011) breaks down the components of self-compassion into three parts: recognition of our common humanity, self-kindness and mindfulness.

Psychoeducation is key to helping people realize they are not alone in their experiences. When I tell clients that picking and pulling are common and explain more about it, they recognize themselves not to be freaks but to be coping the way others have coped; the fog of shame begins to dissipate. Breath work helps with mindfulness and awareness of deeper feelings, and self-kindness develops throughout this process.

The first phase in action

Let's return to Maria. In the following sessions, we went through the process of shaking off shame and replacing it with self-compassion. First, I helped her to see that her hair pulling has been a coping mechanism, not just an enemy.

To make this connection, I asked her to imagine a stress cup somewhere inside of her body. This cup is already pretty full and fills up from the stress she experiences during any given day. Sometimes, when the cup is full of stress, the urges to pick or pull are intense. This is why sometimes, despite her best efforts, she just ends up pulling. I suggested that if we work on relieving some of the stresses that fill her internal cup, she urges to pick or pull may become more manageable. In this way, we can shift to a more compassionate attitude. Instead of asking "What is wrong with me?" she can ask, "What do I need right now? What is my body communicating?"

Maria felt reassured by these ideas. She remembered how much she had to cope with as a teenager. We talked more about her experiences at home and at school at the time of her parents' divorce. She could see that hair pulling fit in as a way to cope, and she was able to cry and be comforted by me. The seeds of self-kindness were planted.

In the next session, Maria was ready to talk about the details of her hair-pulling behavior. She described running her fingers through her hair and searching for kinky hairs, either while she was working or while relaxing and watching TV.

When I listed some of the typical sensory elements of hair pulling, she talked about enjoying finding a hair bulb, looking at it, pulling it off and then chewing on the hair bulb and chewing up and swallowing the hair itself. Again, she laughed nervously and asked me if I knew why people do something so weird as eating their hair.

I let her know that from what I have learned from many clients, pleasure from the chewing sensation tends to be related to the need to release unexpressed anger. She immediately connected with that idea and expressed relief, then told me about all the anger she had to hold in when, 3 years after the divorce, her mother married a man who didn't like children. Her mother put his needs first, and Maria was furious at no longer being the priority. She would either rage, breaking things and getting grounded for weeks, or tuck her anger away to get along in the family.

As we talked through these experiences, Maria's body physically relaxed. This is how co-regulation begins.

Through this process, Maria has gradually shaken off most of her shame and replaced it with self-kindness. Her psychic skin is much sturdier, and she has begun to develop a new sense of self. She has been able to locate and talk through some of the feelings that had gotten locked away in her body. We have settled into a positive alliance and have set some seeds for the skills she will develop in the next phase: exploration and skill-building.

References

Brown, B. (2007). *I thought it was just me (but it isn't): Making the journey from "what will people think?" to "I am enough"*. New York, NY: Gotham Books.

Courtois, C., & Ford, J. (2013). *Treatment of complex trauma: A sequenced, relationship-based approach*. New York, NY: Guilford Press.

Flores, P. (2004). *Addiction as an attachment disorder*. Oxford, UK: Jason Aronson.

Jones, B., Keuthen, N., & Greenberg, E. (2018). Assessment and treatment of trichotillomania (hair pulling disorder) and excoriation (skin picking) disorder. *Clinics in Dermatology, 36*, 728–736.

Main., M. (1991). Metacognitive knowledge, metacognitive monitoring, and singular vs. multiple models of attachment. In C. Parks et al. (Eds.), *Attachment across the life cycle*. London: Routledge.

Miller, W., & Rollnick, S. (2013). *Motivational interviewing: Helping people change* (3rd ed.). New York, NY: The Guilford Press.

Neff, K. (2011). *Self-compassion: The proven power of being kind to yourself*. New York, NY: William Morrow.

Summers, R. (2018). The psychodynamic formulation updated. *American Journal of Psychotherapy, 57*(1), 39–51.

Summers, R., & Barber, J. (2003). Therapeutic alliance as a measurable psychotherapy skill. *Academic Psychiatry, 27*(3), 160–165.

Ziv-Beiman, S. (2015). Integrative psychotherapy and coping with psychopathological syndromes: Dilemmas around the treatment of a patient with resistant trichotillomania. *Journal of Psychotherapy Integration, 25*(3), 175–182.

6   The exploration and skill-building phase

Exploration and skill-building

It is impossible to condense the framework for the entire exploration and skill-building phase into one chapter. Psychodynamic techniques cannot be learned from a manual. I learned to be an effective psychotherapist through ongoing participation in my own individual and group psychotherapy, and in both individual and group consultations.

The safety phase enables the shift into the exploration and skill-building phase. Just like the securely attached toddler, my clients and I now have a secure foundation. This connection between us allows our process to deepen.

Embodied narrative therapy

Many theorists have created helpful books and training manuals that teach therapists how to be emotionally and somatically in the room with each individual. Diana Fosha's (2000) accelerated experiential-dynamic psychotherapy is a model that captures some critical elements of the therapist's stance, including the importance of tracking the client's affect in the room and checking in with a client's nonverbal as well as verbal communications. Peter Levine's seminal 1997 book, *Waking the Tiger*, a helpful introduction to the somatic experiencing modality, is especially useful in releasing the grip of trauma symptoms.

What these approaches have in common is that they connect narrative with emotions and somatic experiences, all versions of what I think of as embodied narrative therapy. Percy & Paré (2021) elucidate the way that new narratives can be created through this process. When we can sit with our clients in the transference and countertransference process, we have the opportunity to help them shake off the ways negative experiences have shaped their sense of self. "Our identities are understood as storied, and the task at hand is to wrest our identities back from normative accounts that

DOI: 10.4324/9781003299097-9

judge us negatively . . . In narrative therapy, the process of reducing suffering is the process of re-authoring" (p. 6).

Joining and mirroring continue to be important connective tissue. This can be on a verbal level but also happens through connecting our nervous systems, the therapist being attuned to pain points of affect that will benefit from slowing down the process. Translating body language into words is a key element of the storytelling in this phase. If my client's hand goes to her hair or skin, or if another physical motion cues me to something left unsaid, I will pause our conversation to explore what feelings may be lurking under the surface. I often ask what a restless body part is communicating, what it would say if it could talk. We check in with our bodies. We process together with the feelings that arise. We breathe.

Exploration: processing the psychodynamic formulation

From a psychodynamic framework, exploration is the working through of the case formulation, paying attention to the dance of transference and countertransference in the therapy room. Adaptive emotional regulation skills are woven into the therapeutic process, with a variety of tools to access the unconscious and get to the root of stubborn resistances.

Ziv-Beiman (2015) illustrated how interpretive work around the psychodynamic case formulation could be applied specifically to understanding and working with trichotillomania. In a case study, she described helping Dana understand the connection between her experience of multigenerational grief and trauma and to release some of the perfectionism that helped her to cope with her parents' fragility. During the treatment, Ziv-Beiman honored Dana's resistance to changing her hair-pulling behavior, focused on building her self-esteem and helped her to separate from her role as the identified patient in the family. She explains how cognitive restructuring was woven into the dynamic work,

> In addition to ongoing interpretive work and active efforts to increase Dana's self-esteem, I actively challenged some of the emotional and cognitive tenets I identified as underlying her distress. These included her belief that she had to disguise the fact that she was helpless and that she needed help in finding the only right way to do things.
>
> (p. 179)

Tools for skill-building

Art therapy is a specific therapeutic modality, and I am not a certified art therapist. However, I have learned from my clients who are drawn to express themselves through art that inviting art into the therapy room can offer a way to symbolize emotions and experiences that may be inexpressible (Holmes, 2001). Images can help to uncover memories and meanings that reside just outside conscious awareness, some of which are triggering the repetitive behaviors.

A whiteboard can serve this function too. For example, Eva, an 11-year-old Caucasian female, was very insistent in her sessions that she was a bad person and not worthy of love. Eva's negative self-talk was so engrained she believed it completely. I handed her the whiteboard to draw what her self-talk would look like if it were a picture, and she drew a large spiky "poison tree." When I asked if any part of her cared for herself, she drew a small, thin sapling. This exercise helped her understand the consequences of continuing to invest in her self-hatred. It also gave me a follow-up reference, to ask her how the little sapling was doing.

Skill #1: emotional expression and modulation

In this stage, I look to broaden the range of emotional expression in therapy, focusing particularly on what are deemed "negative feelings," like jealousy or hatred. I gently challenge the perfectionism defense and get to the feelings underneath each individual's pleasant front. I am mindful that the over-compliance of pickers and pullers tends to manifest as deference to the therapist. I lean in during this part of treatment, as I realize that I am encouraging them to do the thing that scares them the most: being honest about their negative feelings.

Emotional modulation is the ability to choose how to respond to stressful situations rather than act impulsively. The ability to decide how to react is one of the fundamental keys to managing life's difficulties. If we can learn to ask the question "What does my body need?" when urges to pick or pull are high, we can begin to make choices about how to handle those urges. Learning to express our needs to others helps us to build healthy relationships.

Anna, a 35-year-old Jewish woman and mother of two young children, came to see me because of long-standing low self-esteem due to her untreated skin picking and its effects. She had been through the skinpick. com treatment program, and it made her realize she needed to find a therapist, to work through some deeper issues from her past. She saw me weekly for 8 months. I discuss the successful outcome of our work in Chapter 9.

As she narrated her life, Anna talked about how she started picking her skin as a teenager alone in her room, to cope with negative feelings such as sadness and anger. From early childhood she had realized that she could get a lot of positive attention by getting perfect grades and performing as a dancer. She remembers being in a popular crowd but often feeling insecure.

Anna described having a happy childhood. However, her mom had made it clear that some emotions were taboo to express, including rage. Anna felt ashamed of having those bad feelings and she pushed them away.

Currently, a lot of Anna's energy went into self-criticism about how she could sometimes lose her temper as a parent.

Anna's self-criticism, or anger turned inward, was the focus of my interventions. Again, we had to shake off this self-attack and build a compassionate framework.

Often, when I am looking to shift negative self-talk and build self-compassion, a whiteboard is a particularly helpful cognitive tool, and for Anna it was a natural fit, as she liked to journal and draw between our sessions. In one session, she talked about hating that she had picked her face the day before and hated how ugly her skin looked as a result. I used the board to create room for a shift in perspective. I started with her statement, "I hate my picking," and created another category: "What needs is my picking meeting?"

As we talked, I wrote down her answers to the question. She was able to break down the ways her skin picking helped her cope with a variety of circumstances, including when she was annoyed at her kids, when she was anxious about something and when she was sad.

I hate my picking	What needs is my picking meeting?
	• Calms me
	• Releases stress
	• Gets me a break from the kids
	• Distracts me from sad feelings

Anna explained the impact of this exercise in her 3-month follow-up interview:

> I realized that I use picking for a lot of different things! Sometimes I would just use it to stall, and so my husband was waiting for me and I was picking, but I realized that really I just needed to ask him for a few minutes alone before going out as a family.

When finding herself planted at the bathroom mirror, Anna began to ask herself what her body might be telling her about what she needed. She could then modulate her emotions, asking for what she needed instead of impulsively picking. With access to a variety of ways to express and release feelings, it became much easier to make healthier behavioral choices.

This intervention involved cognitive restructuring, but its effectiveness relied on the therapeutic alliance. Because I saw Anna's picking differently than she saw her own behavior, with a wide, compassionate lens, she could start to drop her attachment to the self-attack and connect with my more compassionate appraisal.

Skill #2: processing grief and trauma

In the assessment phase, I make note of precipitating factors involving unresolved grief and/or trauma, and in this phase, we return to those stories (Courtois & Ford, 2013).

When we naturally cycle back to talking about the loss of an attachment figure, perhaps around the time of the client's first engagement with picking or pulling, I encourage them to share their experiences with death and loss while being connected to their bodies and their breath and their emotions. I ask them to tell me about the moments that have stayed in their memories. These may include details like the moment when they learned a health diagnosis or the shock of a sudden loss, any medical trauma, a funeral or reactions to anniversaries.

In this way, clients can finally grieve the losses they pushed away earlier in their lives, when they didn't have anyone to help them contain and accept the depth of their feelings. Once grief has been processed and released from the body, often through tears, new possibilities may open. In later sessions, clients often come across positive memories of their loved ones that had been obscured by the memory of their loss.

Processing trauma involves getting rid of the emotional and physiological residue of the experience. The only way to resolve the need for dissociation and avoidance strategies is to reconnect trauma-related emotions, body reactions, thoughts and consequences. Courtois and Ford (2013) explain: "Emotion processing enables the client to safely experience and appraise in present time the physical sensations, emotions and thoughts that he or she had interpreted as signals of overwhelming danger and associated powerlessness after the trauma" (p. 151).

Skill #3: assertiveness and communication

Anger is an adaptive emotion, designed to help people set boundaries (Greenberg & Paivio, 1997). When anger isn't expressed, it has to go somewhere. If it is turned inward, it becomes a force of aggressive energy. Hair pulling and skin picking are to some degree an expression of this energy building up, and being let out, bit by bit. Many different feelings get internalized, but anger lights the fire of other internal chaos.

Frustration is the main feeling my clients face once we peel back the layers of perfection. In order to foster their ability to know and express their needs, set boundaries and speak up, I start by helping them share these with me. A good time for this is when I can tell that a client is frustrated with me. There are so many things my clients can be mad at me about! I am imperfect – I say the wrong thing and ask too many questions. Putting their angry feelings into words can take pressure off my clients' urges to pick and pull.

The ability to express anger directly is a key assertiveness skill, and it helps us to set boundaries that keep us safe. Often, my clients have experienced being hurt or taken advantage of as a result of their determination to be nice at all costs. This niceness involves disengaging from the awareness of frustration building in the body.

Encouraging aggression toward ourselves as therapists is easier said than done. We have to grapple with the desire to be liked, our own fear of conflict, our insecurities about our skills. I find it very helpful to remember that the aggressive energy in my clients' bodies needs to be moved out. The more they can express their dissatisfaction with me, the better they will learn that their anger doesn't have to be toxic. This process, in turn, will help clients set boundaries in their relationships. Once they realize it is possible to express anger and frustration without destroying their relationships, they can begin to share a wider range of feelings in all their interactions with others.

For example, I ask Sara, a young adult who has been in treatment for skin picking for a few months, why she hasn't mentioned that I started our session a few minutes late (I am usually very punctual). She says she understands and isn't upset about it. I note that she hasn't been looking at me during the session and that her hands seem very restless. I remind her that if she can express all her feelings, it will help me get to know her. I wonder aloud what her hands might be saying.

Finally, she tells me that her hands want to scratch at her skin. I note that the energy in her hands is being misdirected, as she is probably mad at me. Tears well up behind her eyes and she tells me that I hurt her feelings when she sat on my waiting-room couch, wondering if I forgot about her. Then I apologize for running late, repairing the rupture in our connection. She can now relax with me in a way she hadn't yet been able to do.

As Sara learns how to read the emotional cues in her body and to share these emotions in relationships, she can begin to assert herself more in the world. This in turn brings her more self-confidence and helps her draw boundaries in her relationships.

Skill #4: sublimation

Sublimation, the channeling of aggressive energy into productive activities, is one way to release the extra energy in the hands of pickers and pullers, without doing harm to the self or others. One form of sublimation is engagement in boxing (see the Introduction for my own story), with frustration literally transferring from the hands to a heavy bag. Martial arts, running or engaging in creative activities can also release aggressive energy.

Once there is a way to release frustration from the body, softer comforts become more appealing. Healthy grooming can bring a different energy to engaging with the skin and nails. When biting the cuticles is the go-to behavior, nail care and manicures can provide a different element of sensory input. Hair care can feel comforting and increase confidence. Choices around cuts and colors can provide different ways to think about hair, which can lead to a shift from criticism of one's appearance to enjoyment of self-expression.

The next stage of soft comforts is inviting in healthy relationships, or strengthening existing relationships, so that partners can help soothe partners. I am always amazed to watch that part of my clients' growth: when they find and maintain healthier relationships. Group therapy often comes in as an adjunct in this growth process.

Case example: Elizabeth

Elizabeth, a high-achieving, bisexual Caucasian woman in her mid-thirties, entered individual and, later, group therapy with me to work through the negative relationship patterns she seemed to repeat. She had a very healthy therapeutic alliance with a therapist in a different state and had recovered from an eating disorder. She was being treated for major depression by a psychiatrist.

We started our work together in 2008. In 2022, at the time of this writing, Elizabeth and I were coming to the adjournment stage of our relationship. She planned to move out of state shortly, leaving biweekly individual therapy and a weekly group of which she was a participant since its founding in 2015. She liked the idea of participating in an interview to review our work together over the years, through ups and downs, and we were both moved by the process. This vignette is mostly focused on her individual work with me through the exploration phase, as aided at times by her work in the group.

Elizabeth explained why she sought treatment with me about a year after she had moved to Austin, "I was just in a job that was awful, and I felt sad all of the time. And I was just desperate because I had that feeling of being stuck." She was also in a dead-end relationship and experiencing a depressive episode.

She didn't seek me out for my expertise in BFRBs, although she did have a very specific body-focused behavior: pressing into, biting or ripping at the skin on her fingers, especially her thumbs. She explains why that behavior wasn't a focus of therapy for her, and why, in fact, she would have rejected direct attempts to get rid of it,

> I guess it really wasn't an issue for me. It had gotten to the point where I could allow the rest of my nails to grow out, and just pick at my thumbs, and I could keep those hidden for the most part. So, it was something I had no desire to change.

One element that was important to her in the safety phase was the establishment of clear boundaries. "I feel a great sense of security, where there's no nebulousness around this relationship. I feel like it's a very close, warm relationship, and I trust her so much, and I feel it's a very secure, safe place." This security set the stage for us to move deeper into some of the internal pain she had carried throughout the years.

I developed a case formulation to make sense of her use of her thumb hurting to regulate her emotions. As described in Chapter 2, Elizabeth was the youngest of four children, the two oldest were half-brothers and her sister was 6 years older than her. The group of them was more than a handful for her overtaxed and overworked parents. As I got to know her life story, I learned that she held deep shame and pain about being sexually abused as a child, that her other siblings had very loud ways of expressing their pain, and she was relegated to being the one who had it together. She was largely out of touch with her body, as it held unbearable trauma residue, and we realized that her coping mechanisms all involved being in charge of the sensations she felt, rather than being at the mercy of invasive thoughts and feelings. Elizabeth explains,

> I just know that whenever I felt really upset or emotional, I would just pick at myself, or bite my nails or something like that. For me, as far as really causing pain to myself, whether picking or an eating disorder or compulsive exercise, that was definitely a reaction of wanting control of my body. It was like "I will cause my body pain. No one else is allowed. I will control what my body is doing." And I think that was all a reaction to being sexually abused as a kid.

During our first years together, I watched Elizabeth develop a healthier relationship with food, gain confidence, re-engage in art and form some new friendships. Still, she continued to find herself in a submissive role in romantic relationships. Additionally, she remained resistant to expressing her anger, and I could usually only tell when she was angry at me or someone in the group when she would engage in her go-to nonverbal communication, pressing on the side of her thumb with two fingers or biting on the skin around the nail, sometimes drawing blood.

At first, I tried to comment directly on her pressing and biting behaviors in group or individual sessions, to no effect. Elizabeth would use a death glare to communicate her resistance to exploring the behaviors. I experienced frustration toward her at these times, but it was at a level that I could notice the feeling, sit with the frustration and be aware that I was holding a lot of unexpressed frustration for Elizabeth. I knew that I needed not to erupt in anger at her as her father had done when he was angry at her sister, teaching her to stay out of the mix, or ignore her veiled aggression like her mother had done. As Flores (2004) explains this process,

> The therapist's job is not to deny the emotional responses evoked in him, nor is it his job to allow himself to be induced to repeat the old patterns. Rather; his task is to alter his responses so that a new and different outcome can be achieved.
>
> (157)

Joining Elizabeth's resistance to exploring the aggressive energy in her hands, I shifted to studying possible triggers for it within interactions in the group. In one session, I noticed that although Elizabeth had been pressing on her finger consistently, when she began to talk, the behavior stopped. When she disengaged from the conversation, she went back to the pressing. The longer she went without giving her input into a conversation, the more intensely she would engage in the behavior.

In our individual session later in the week, I mentioned to Elizabeth what I had noticed about the connection between holding in her feelings in group and pressing on her nail. She acknowledged that she had been very frustrated with the group, who were all staying on the surface of things and not talking about the things that really bothered them. This opened up what she called the "rage phase" of our work, where she felt free to tell me how incredibly disappointing I was as a therapist, and how I could never help her get any better, and maybe therapy was only making her worse. Once, in group, she said that a question I asked was "SO STUPID!" While bristling at the word stupid, I was able to enjoy Elizabeth's rebellion. I observed a touch of childish glee in her eyes and a pout on her mouth. My body softened as I realized that she sounded very much like a child, trying out a mean phrase in a way that was hostile yet vulnerable.

Elizabeth explained that it was only the quality of our relationship that got us through the times these rage years.

> There were years, full years where I felt like absolutely nothing was happening. I would say 'This isn't working, this is pointless. I'm

wasting money.' And I would still stay, because I trusted Stacy, even though I was mad most of the time. I thought it was dumb, but I would stay. And I think for me, that feels like an essential part of therapy, is to trust the therapist enough to stay even when you think it is stupid.

After that, she felt freer to talk about being angry about lots of things, and at lots of people in her current life and in her past. We talked through how furious she had been at her parents and her siblings growing up and always feeling like she had to take care of herself, and how she never felt safe enough to express her rage. She was able to talk through some of her most painful experiences and connect the feelings, memories, sensations and emotions that had gone underground. In the process, she recognized that she had disconnected from any sense of her legs at an early age, rarely experiencing any sense of being grounded. We cried together for her little self. She described this period as a very difficult but important part of our work together,

> I remember when I was a child, I was a deeply angry child, and I went to a psychiatrist when I was six and he told my parents that I was a very angry child. And my parents were like, "No, she's not, she cries a lot, she's sad." And so by the time I saw Stacy I was convinced I was a person who just didn't have anger. And then, with her, things transitioned, and I just became a burning ball of rage, it was all-consuming, and then I was able to have room for other feelings.

Three years ago, Elizabeth was ready to date again after the end of an unfulfilling relationship. She noticed that she was dating differently, actually enjoying the process. She attributes this change to having gained a sense of agency the more she used her voice to express her feelings and assert her needs with me and with the group. She explains,

> In the past, relationships felt scary, because I'd get in a situation, and I'd feel like I had no capacity to get out. But a few years ago, something happened that felt like magic, where suddenly, I felt like I had agency in my life. And that became the realization that changed everything, that moment where I realized, "I am not a child, I am an adult person, and I get to make my own choices and have that agency."

At this point in her life, stuck is definitely not a feeling Elizabeth would use to describe her experience. In fact, after meeting a kind life partner and marrying him, she has found a new job. They are moving to a place she really wants to live, buying their first home together.

She described her experience in therapy as a re-authoring of her story, "I think therapy really helped me to be an actual coherent, cohesive person that had this narrative throughout my entire life, and I could put all of the pieces of my narrative and myself back together." Along the way, she also developed a sense of choice about whether to engage in thumb hurting, "Now I have that awareness of what's happening and why, and I can choose to do it or not."

Elizabeth points to the significance of including her body in the process of healing and sublimating her aggression, both in my office and in outside endeavors,

> One thing we did early on is Stacy got me to think about putting my feet on the ground, and it's something I'm not good at. I like to hug my feet. But I started to take a bodywork class that was focused on a lot of stomping. It was amazing how important it was for me just to think about where my feet are and where my legs are, and how much that calmed me, and then allowed me to express more emotion too.

References

Courtois, C., & Ford, J. (2013). *Treatment of complex trauma: A sequenced, relationship-based approach*. New York, NY: Guilford Press.

Flores, P. (2004). *Addiction as an attachment disorder*. Lanham, MD: Jason Aronson, Inc.

Fosha, D. (2000). *The transforming power of affect: A model for accelerated change*. New York, NY: Basic Books.

Greenberg, L., & Paivio, S. (1997). *Working with emotions in psychotherapy*. New York, NY: Guilford Press.

Holmes, J. (2001). *The search for the secure base: Attachment theory and psychotherapy*. New York, NY: Routledge.

Levine, P. (1997). *Waking the tiger: Healing trauma*. Berkeley, CA: North Atlantic Books.

Percy, I., & Paré, D. (2021). Narrative therapy and mindfulness: Intention attention, ethics: Part #1. *Journal of Systemic Therapy*, 40(3), 1–14.

Ziv-Beiman, S. (2015). Integrative psychotherapy and coping with psychopathological syndromes: Dilemmas around the treatment of a patient with resistant trichotillomania. *Journal of Psychotherapy Integration*, 25(3), 175–182.

7 A healing herd

Group psychotherapy to build community

Group support

Given that shame and secrecy are ubiquitous companions to BFRBs, it makes intuitive sense that group support would be an important component of treatment. Neff (2009) lists identification with others as one of the three building blocks of self-compassion. Seeing oneself in others leads to a sense of universality to replace isolation. "Common humanity involves recognizing that all humans are imperfect, fail and make mistakes. [Universality] connects one's own flawed condition to the shared human condition so that greater perspective is taken towards personal shortcomings and difficulties" (p. 212).

To meet this need for common humanity and relief from isolation, the TLC Foundation for BFRBs has founded BFRBD support groups since its inception, maintaining updated listings on their website and connecting people all over the country and internationally. Their annual retreats also serve this purpose – teens and adults can frolic in the swimming pool without concern for wigs or makeup, shaking off shame as they let go of the camouflage. I have led a number of group workshops at TLC Foundation retreats and conferences, and the development of bonds between participants is a key healing factor.

Though the value of group support is evident, few studies have explored the possible benefits of therapist-led group therapy in BFRBD treatment. A 2006 study compared the effectiveness of two kinds of therapist-led groups: skill-building and support groups, each with 12 members. The stated goal of treatment was alleviation of symptoms. Neither group was found to be particularly helpful toward achieving the desired long-term symptom relief (Diefenbach et al., 2006). Research in 2019 comparing support groups with psychodrama groups to treat excoriation disorder, with around 10 members per group, found that both types of groups were effective to the same extent at reducing skin-picking behaviors. This outcome pointed to the peer support element rather than psychodrama as the key change agent (Gulassa et al., 2019). The authors

DOI: 10.4324/9781003299097-10

note that emotional dysregulation was a commonly identified trigger for skin picking and suggest that future groups focus on the enhancement of emotional regulation skills.

Asplund et al. (2021) studied 40 participants in group therapy from a cognitive-behavioral approach enhanced by acceptance and commitment therapy (ACT) techniques found that the groups were successful in reducing behavioral symptoms in the short term. There was an unexplained discrepancy between the participants who struggled with skin picking maintaining their progress after a year, while those struggling with trichotillomania tended to relapse by the time of the 2-month follow-up (Asplund et al., 2021). The authors noted that discrepancy as a subject for future research. Once again, though these results were positive, the focus on symptom relief without an exploration of their roots misses the opportunity to heal attachment-based wounds so relevant to this population.

In a psychodynamic group, though behavioral change is still a goal for most members, the idea of getting rid of symptoms is not at the forefront. Instead, group can help members identify triggers for BFRB urges, thus addressing the underlying emotional dysregulation. The focus of the group is on the relations between members, as they help one another develop a new range of emotional regulation skills. These include awareness and tolerance of feelings, lessening of shame, ability to talk openly about body-focused behaviors with one's peers, development of self-compassion, awareness of triggers, ability to talk about hard feelings like anger, and the discovery of new ways to self-soothe and/or get restless energy out of the body.

For preteens and teens who pick and pull, I have found that groups with a focus on psychoeducation along with emotional, behavioral and social skill-building are a good fit. These are supportive groups rather than process groups, with members providing validation and gentle questioning without engaging in deep interpersonal exploration. Research shows that one key developmental task of adolescence is to find a place to belong and feel good about oneself, and preteens and teens in my groups have certainly gained confidence from being around peers who share similar struggles (Ragilienė, 2016).

When I ask teen clients to imagine what it will be like to be in an issue-focused group for people with BFRBDs, they worry that it will be a group full of weird and unhappy people. Upon meeting one another, they tend to experience relief that their peers actually seem pretty normal, except that they too pick and pull. This commonality and friendship helps them shake off a layer of shame and secrecy from the start.

In those 8–10-week groups, I loosely focus each group session on a topic. This gives group members a chance to connect around common experiences, such as whether they keep their behaviors secret from family and friends, how they handle pool parties and dating, what happens if someone points out a bald spot or scab, and how they react depending on whether the comment is kind or cruel. Once members hear their own stories reflected in those of their peers, they begin to feel compassion for one another and for themselves. Through psychoeducation and conversation, they learn that they have common emotional stressors that lead to similar behaviors, which in turn helps them to better identify and express their feelings.

Ivy was 16 when she began weekly therapy with me. A Caucasian female, she found me after trying to get help for her skin picking from several other therapists. About a year into my work with her, I started a new group for teens struggling with BFRBs. I asked if she would be interested in joining the group and she was on board within a minute. Ivy described that moment in an interview 12 years after we ended our work together,

> Once Stacy said that there with other girls who also had dermatillomania or trichotillomania, I was like, "I'm sorry. What? When can I meet them?" It's like the world opened up for me. And I was like, "Yes, let's do it."

Returning to the parallel research on animals with BFRBs that showed improvement in symptoms when a companion was added to the pen, group therapy can be one way to find a herd, or a community, to belong to. Group connection can help members meet some of the needs for comfort that are met by picking and pulling behaviors. Natterson-Horowitz and Bowers (2013) imagined this possibility of a healing herd for people on the self-harm continuum, originally mentioning cutters, but applicable here, "Like a lonely horse reintroduced to a herd, isolated [hair pullers] could be encouraged to find herds of their own" (p. 224).

This is the realm of change therapist-led groups can engender, as the therapist facilitates healthy attachments to peers and social development can get back on track. The benefits of working on emotional regulation skills in the social playground are immense. These new attachments can lead to changes in the brain. Yalom and Leszcz (2020) reflected on therapy groups: "New relational experience may foster neurobiological changes by activating neural pathways . . . The neurobiological impacts may even have the potential to repair the individual's genetic substrate damaged by early life adversity" (p. 70, footnote).

Ivy explained that one main benefit of group therapy was being with other teens who were like her. She remembers this experience reducing her feelings of shame and isolation,

> I remember just sharing our experiences, how the picking has been. And just hearing the details from other girls that I was afraid to share

was just so empowering. I was like, "Okay, if they can talk about it so can I. And there's nothing wrong with it or scary about it."

The group did create a sense of universality for Ivy, fostering self-compassion,

It just made me feel like this is something that we're all in together, and we're trying to figure out how to make it not so invasive or not affect our lives so much on a daily basis. I just remember after every session I felt like a weight was lifted.

Other benefits included the development of self-kindness, as Ivy reflected, "Receiving compassion from others and then giving it to the others in the group, that would help me later on feel more kindness and compassion towards myself."

Modern analytic group therapy

For adults, I have found that psychodynamic process groups can expand beyond the support function into the arena of enhancing secure attachment. A literature review in February 2022 on PubMed for the terms psychodynamic group therapy and trichotillomania, skin-picking, hair-pulling and body-focused repetitive behaviors showed that my own 2015 article was the only peer-reviewed paper on the topic (Nakell, 2015). In that article, I explored the ways some group processes are specifically helpful to those who struggle with BFRBs.

I illuminated the way the group process helped members listen to their bodies, voice their feelings and receive validation. Group members also helped one another recognize the impact of traumatic experiences on their emotional development, building self-compassion. Groups give me an in vivo opportunity to help people let go of the perfectionism defense. This, in turn, helps them to build more advanced adaptive emotional regulation skills like managing conflicts and setting healthy boundaries.

Unlike with skill-building and support groups, there is no rule book to guide the group psychotherapist. Group therapy is an art that must be studied and practiced. Organizations such as the American Group Psychotherapy Association and the Center for Group Studies (CGS) provide didactic and experiential training for those who want to run groups, with CGS focusing on training therapists in modern group analysis.

Yalom and Leszcz (2020), in their seminal book on group psychotherapy, identify the working through of family relationships in vivo as key to the group's healing potential:

What is important, though, is not that early familial conflicts are relived, but that they are relived *correctively* . . . For many group members, then, working out problems with therapists and other members is also working through unfinished business from long ago.

(pp. 27–28)

In modern analysis, the power of transference and countertransference is a key element of this work. Modern analytic group techniques are expounded on in the work of Spotnitz, Rosenthal and Ormont. Modern analytic group theory outlines the way a group becomes a representation of the family. Transferences to other members and to the leader bring up old, familiar patterns. The group can help change these tired stories, as the leader encourages new avenues of emotional expression to counter the repression of painful emotional experiences such as rage and grief. As Rosenthal (1996) explains, "the group attains a higher level of emotional development when immature forms of communication are replaced by more mature behaviors" (p. 75).

As in individual treatment, the modern analytic approach brings key elements for working through difficulties specifically with regulating emotions and developing intimate connections with others. Ormont (2001) described the development of a group from the first stage to later stages: bringing resistances into play, working to resolve the fears that underlie these resistances and identifying early forms of intimacy to allow more mature intimacy to develop. Modern analytic techniques such as the group contract, use of immediacy, joining and mirroring, bridging, and drawing aggression toward the leader help the group therapist to move the group through these stages.

Joining a group

The clients I invite into a group have already developed a relationship with me, either through working with me individually or going through a group intake process. I coordinate with their individual therapist when indicated. In individual therapy, the client has begun to develop the beginnings of a more solid self beneath the shell of the "good girl" or "good boy," building a healthier emotional buffer between the self and the world. We have attended to young parts of the self, working on basic skills such as mindfulness, self-compassion and distress tolerance.

At some point in my individual treatment with a person who is suffering from a BFRBD, I evaluate whether that person will benefit from group. I will begin to notice that a client is better able to calm down when dysregulated. They have gotten more in touch with their internal signals and can take deep breaths as they talk through difficult feelings. We've done some processing of grief and trauma, and I feel like I know their story: what led to their picking or pulling, what triggers current episodes, where they struggle and what topics bring up their defenses. When I notice that we have been talking a lot about a lack of intimacy in their lives, or difficulty standing up for themselves in work conflicts or forming a sense of community, I begin to check in about whether group therapy might be a good next step in our process.

The group contract

To guide pre-group preparation, Ormont (2001) introduced the tool of the group contract. The contract consists of a set of agreements about group participation, to provide structure and investigate likely areas of resistance even before the first group session. When the client is preparing to join the group, we spend several sessions going over the contract carefully. Agreements include arriving at each session on time, maintaining confidentiality, taking one's fair share of the group time, paying on time, not socializing outside group, and putting thoughts and feelings into words instead of actions.

This last agreement is the one that is likely to bring up the most resistance from pickers and pullers. The idea of expressing thoughts and feelings honestly at the moment in a group runs counter to all the defenses people with BFRBDs have invested in throughout their lives – putting on a happy face, accommodating and pleasing others, and avoiding conflict.

At the same time, therapists should be aware that group therapy is sure to bring up group members' resistance in full force. For someone who struggles with BFRBs, this means staying on the surface of emotions and trying to smooth out potential conflicts. It is important to support these defenses for quite some time in a new group, as members will need to employ their usual avoidance strategies to keep from getting overwhelmed.

When I talk through the contract with a potential new member, I try to set the scene for what they will experience. I explain that when one brings together a therapist and a group of people, transformative things happen. I might say something like,

> Somehow someone in the group will remind you of your sister, or your mother, or your partner. Whatever happens in your relationships in the world will somehow show up in the group room, and we will be able to talk about the things that get in the way of you developing better relationships. The group is the place where we put words to the thoughts we have about one another, the annoyances and affections that usually go unsaid.

I remind prospective group members that it will be challenging, and that feelings of anxiety and excitement are a normal and appropriate reaction.

Bridging

At its most basic, bridging is the group therapist's way of connecting members with one another. In Ormont's (2001) words, "the term *bridging* refers to any technique designed to strengthen emotional connections between members, or to develop connections where they did not exist before" (p. 264).

When the group becomes cohesive, bridging becomes more complex, as group members can help one another name feelings they too have tucked away out of sight. Ormont explained, "By bridging, we bring out similarities in feeling tones, in history, and in aspiration between members, and help them recognize capacities for understanding that they did not know they possessed" (p. 277).

For example, I might ask a quiet person about someone who has been quiet: "Joe, why do you think Amanda has been quiet tonight?" Joe might say she looks sad. Amanda might agree, and even if not, she might talk more about what she is feeling. Just as I have helped them put words to body language in our individual work, now other group members begin to help one another with that translation. A member may find herself asking a group member whose foot is incessantly tapping, "What does your foot need to say?"

Leader drawing aggression toward herself

As in individual therapy, this modern analytic group technique is the one many therapists find the most challenging: the therapist draws aggression toward herself. In groups, therapists face unique countertransference resistance, as being called out by a client in front of a group can bring on self-attack and shame and it is easy to feel deskilled.

As Morris (2021) explained, female therapists must resolve resistances to experiencing and therapeutically working with anger in order to meet the aggression that comes their way. She pointed out that female archetypes from fairy tales do not work effectively with aggression,

> Cinderella, the Wicked Queen, and Glinda all had problems with aggression . . . The Queen's feelings and impulses are never respected as the aggression that lives in all of us . . . so the lesson in this tale is to split them off and deny them.
>
> (p. 114)

Aggressive energy needs to be released from the body. Modern analysts work with the understanding that aggressive energy, if not discharged outwardly, gets turned upon the self. The aim of individual and group treatment is to reverse the process of turning aggression on the self (what Spotnitz termed the *narcissistic defense*) and direct this energy outward in constructive ways (Spotnitz & Nagelberg 1960). For those with BFRBs, the more pent-up frustration becomes, the likelier it is to be expressed indirectly as steam, angry and hostile, doing damage to the self and/or others. If a client can let out their fury at me about something I did wrong, I can offer a reparative experience by meeting them in that space. I can help them to convert angry energy into words. By understanding the frustrated need behind the outburst we have a better chance of playing it out differently the next time.

In order to help group members turn their aggressive energy on me, I have had to reckon with my difficulty navigating my own tendency to turn anger on myself for making mistakes. Several weeks into my first therapy group in my private practice, I sat, stunned, when a group member, after describing a manic moment, got up and turned the lights in my office off and on and off and then back on, and sat back down.

I remember being frozen and making a joke about how she was "determined to make us experience her world!" When the group was over, I called my consultant sobbing and feeling like a failure for letting a group member take over the group space. She helped me regain my footing as we talked about my reaction, and I was able to process the incident with the group the following week. The group member was sullen and quiet, and other group members were able to turn their anger on me for failing to keep the space safe. I acknowledged that it I had allowed the group member to break our agreement to stay in our seats and talk about our feelings rather than act them out. To my surprise, the group didn't fall apart that day, and I learned how to help group members metabolize their frustration more effectively.

Understanding that I don't need to take the aggression turned my way personally, I can use myself as a reparative attachment figure to help clients release frustrations that have been stuck inside for too long. Once group members understand that I welcome their negative feelings, it's easy for them to find fault with the way I am leading the group. I have so many rules! I ask them to feel awful feelings! We talk about uncomfortable things! Recently, in the times of COVID-19, we've moved online. It's not fair! It's frustrating!

As group members feel freer to express their irritation without retaliation or abandonment from me, they begin to relax in the room in ways they were unable to while growing up. Again, co-regulation begets better self-regulation, and this time, we have the opportunity to work through sibling conflicts and undeveloped social skills, to continue to strengthen the psychic skin and build emotional insulation. The dance of transference and countertransference between group members and me, as well as among members, helps loosen the grip of the perfection defense.

Fiddle toys

For those who pick and pull, I have incorporated fiddle toys as a soft comfort to calm the central nervous system in place of the hard comfort of picking and pulling, at least in my office. For those group members who don't pick or pull, I explain that sometimes fiddle toys can be helpful to keep the hands busy, and that they can even help the group translate feelings into words. In this way, I set the stage for the mutual understanding of a tool that is less commonly used in therapy groups.

In a process group, with the emphasis on putting thoughts and feelings into words, use of any object to occupy the hands is usually discouraged. As with drinking or eating in the room, the idea is that any behavior besides talking will dilute verbal emotional expression.

However, the need to "fiddle" is very real for this population. Since I am asking that they not engage in picking or pulling behaviors when feeling emotionally overwhelmed, in my group room – as in individual therapy – fiddle toys can serve as transitional objects, providing another way to soothe the central nervous system as the clients begin to find words for their feelings.

Though we may have successfully substituted fiddle toys for touching skin and hair in individual sessions, we need to revisit this agreement for group therapy. I remind clients that if I see their hands moving toward their skin or hair during a group session, I will ask that they take one of the fiddle toys. That way, they can get the restless energy out of their bodies, and we can investigate what feelings from the group process may have led their hands to need to fiddle.

It is important to be flexible and open to the ways fiddle toys may be used in the group, both to communicate and, at times, to avoid communication. Some members might use them to calm their nervous systems through awkward moments or to express their creativity. However, if I see that a group member is zoning out while playing with a fiddle toy, I might ask the member to put it aside to break the trance and bring her back into the room. Some group members may fiddle with something each time we meet, while others may outgrow the toys as they improve their communication skills.

Case example: working through resistances

The group featured here has been ongoing since 2014. The first vignette begins with the founding of the group. In the following vignettes, between 2019 and 2022, no original members remain. The overlap between past and current group members has led to the development and maintenance of group norms over time.

Early in my career, I began a group with only three members. I have room for six in my office and have enjoyed keeping groups small, though my online groups now allow for eight members. Six people had signed up, and they had a variety of presenting issues and were diverse in other ways, including race and gender. Three decided the group wasn't for them as the time got closer, and the three who showed up that day all struggled with BFRBs. They shared many other similarities. All were heterosexual Caucasian women in their late twenties to early thirties, all had similar family structures, even including a history that included a mean older sibling, and they connected right away in the group room. Elise was the lone skin picker in the group, and the others were hair pullers.

The similarities included comparable defenses that led to unique challenges, especially being very nice to one another and having superficial conversation. Elise tended to be open with her expressions of annoyance and was emotionally "messier" than the others, who tended to be polite at all costs but could talk about being sad. All preferred to avoid emotions if possible.

Status quo resistance

The first resistance that emerged was the status quo resistance. Rosenthal (1987) defines this resistance:

> Status quo, inertia, or doldrum resistance . . . reflects the feeling that maintenance of their present state of functioning is all that can be asked of them. This is demonstrated in wishes to drift along aimlessly and have a gratifying time together.
>
> (p. 186)

The countertransference resistance I had to work through for most of the first 2 years was my experience of being bored with them. This may sound like a long time, but the modern analytic idea is that the therapy group works as a holding space to process primitive emotional experiences. This work will be slow but can restart the emotional development process that was stymied due to the early difficulties with regulation commonly experienced by those with BFRBDs.

I found quickly that group members' shared coping strategy of burying emotions and presenting a happy face led them to collectively resist moving beyond the emotional surface. For example, one day about 3 months into the group, Tracy described in great detail an elaborate setup to stage a run-in with a man she found attractive, talking for 10 minutes straight. I checked in with Elise, and rather than expressing any of the irritation or boredom I was experiencing, she launched into her own 10-minute parallel experience of staging a run-in with a man. I realized I was the only one feeling frustrated, while the group members were enjoying identifying with one another and avoiding difficult feelings.

At times, I tried to challenge the group's collective sense that one-sided relationships were all they could expect for themselves, and members reacted blankly, with disbelief. I often invited them to direct their anger toward me as an imperfect group leader. Each member would not only deflect my attempts but also support the others in doing so, rendering most of my interventions dead on arrival. My first reaction to this continuing dynamic was to give up on pushing them and to conclude the group was a failure. I wondered whether I had made a mistake in starting the group without more diversity among members, as they seemed only to boost one another's resistance to change. I turned to my consultant often to process my boredom and frustration. Only with that discharge could I allow group members the space to resist change until they were ready to proceed.

As new norms are created in a group, members begin to reflect on their barriers to emotional expression. This ability to witness their social selves in action is called mentalization. Mentalization creates room for a choice. Instead of reaching for hair, nails or skin, group members can try on healthier behaviors.

Two years into the group process, Elise finally put into words the group's resistance: "We make it so hard for you! We don't like talking about our feelings, so we put up a force field to keep you from getting to them."

Compliance resistance

Once group members identify their defenses, there is room to develop new norms that upend some of these rules about squelching feelings and presenting as "perfect" at all costs. The group begins to solidify and form a different, more connected space where feelings are put into words.

In the next iteration of the group, we tackled the perfectionism defense more deeply. Ormont (2001) terms this complying and defines it as an attitudinal resistance,

> Doing the "right" thing but without any underlying spirit . . . We must understand that to the patient these defenses feel successful. They're second nature, they help him survive . . . He will need much help before he can acknowledge on a gut level the existence of these defenses, their power, their function, and the fantasies that fuel them.
>
> (p. 89)

Ormont suggests that we turn to group members to help each other become aware of these sticky resistances.

At the time of these vignettes, the group was full with six members and was much more diverse than the original group, in presenting both issues and demography, as I had originally hoped. The group included three members of Middle Eastern backgrounds, two males and a female. One of the males was in America on a work visa; the others were first-generation Americans. Two female members were Caucasian, both liberal with conservative parents, and the other was Mexican American. Group members were of mixed sexual orientations and a number of the members described themselves as gender fluid.

Amal was a first-generation lesbian Middle Eastern American who picked her skin. She identified as a perfectionist. The only female in a set of triplets, she joined the group shortly after graduating from college. She felt a lot of pressure to be successful, both in her own family and in her chosen path toward social justice – two goals that often came into tension. Her skin picking came to the fore in adolescence, when she was struggling with how to find a sense of belonging in a largely white neighborhood and school. Amal's picking was focused, as she obsessed about small imperfections on her skin and sometimes felt reluctant to go out due to picking and its aftermath.

Ari was a shy and sweet bisexual, male college student on the gender continuum who defined himself as a first-generation Palestinian American. His mother was Muslim, his father was a secular Muslim, and Ari identified somewhere in the middle. He had sought treatment with me for other impulsive and compulsive behaviors, but he did have a history of nail-biting. Ari had, up until that point, expressed only positive feelings toward me, even after I double-booked one of his sessions. When others said they would be mad at me if I double-booked on them, he talked about how anger wasn't welcome in his family, as his father demanded complete obedience from his wife and his children, and how it was hard to even pinpoint angry feelings in his body.

It was very helpful that Amal was able to relate to Ari's experiences of the firm patriarchal dynamics in Middle Eastern families. In different cultures, hair and skin mean different things, and in first-generation Americans, culture clashes can show up in the hatred of ethnic hair, rebellious hairstyles not approved by parents including play around ideas about gender and hair.

Amal had taken to picking up a long plastic caterpillar from the tray at the beginning of the session. At first, she used it to occupy her restless hands and give herself somewhere to look other than at other group members; she touched its feet softly and ran them over her hands. One week, she touched the caterpillar differently, grabbing it from both sides and squeezing it, hard. It caught the attention of another group member, who asked her what she was so mad about. She was able to laugh at how her hands had made obvious her angry feelings, and she talked about how she was starting to get annoyed with the group, as people had been making small talk in the room.

During the next group session, Ari, who had never before interacted with the toy tray, grabbed the same puffy caterpillar before the session began. His first time playing with it, he did what Amal had done – squeezing both sides, hard. I asked him what he was expressing with his hands, and he laughed and said he didn't think he was expressing anything. When I asked Amal if she believed him, she said, "No, I think he's mad at somebody! It might be you – he hasn't looked once at you since we sat down." Ari demurred, "Well, I guess I am mad at you for charging me for missing next week's group session even though it falls on a holiday week."

I asked him to say more.

"It just doesn't seem fair! You're the one who decides which holidays count, and it's random and this time it's really pissing me off!" This opened the conversation to others, who talked about the ways my rules and boundaries seemed unfair, which led to memories about the rules set by their parents. The transference of experiences with their parents onto me allowed us to talk more openly about feelings that once felt unsafe. There was a tangible sense of relief in the room, as Ari finally talked about the anger that builds up inside him and how his hands want to punch things.

Resistance to intimacy

At some point in the last couple of years, I have noticed that members are more open to sharing their feelings as they work through the resistance to intimacy. Ormont (2001) described some of the features of this mature state. Group members make emotional space for each other, feelings are felt in the moment, members are taking emotional risks, and memories of early positive attachments are rediscovered.

Catherine was a heterosexual Caucasian woman in her late twenties who picked her skin. She has difficulty expressing her feelings in intimate relationships, which was related to her parents' painful divorce when she was a preteen. She had a great deal of ambivalence toward her stepfather.

One evening, Catherine gave an update about her stepfather's recent health setback. She let us know it looked like he was going to get better, and she was glad, but was still not happy to have him in her life. The room went uncomfortably quiet. Catherine scratched at her scalp a few times. I asked her what I should understand about the quiet in the room. She said she didn't know, and others chimed in about being tired and not wanting to feel feelings.

"Okay, we don't need to go deep! Let's stay light," I suggested.

Light conversation led to Catherine telling us about her new creative endeavor, making herbal skin remedies at home. There was another, less uncomfortable silence. I noticed that Catherine was rubbing her dress. She was comforting herself in a new, softer way than I had seen before. I noted it aloud and asked if she had a blankie when she was a child. She did and talked happily about that childhood blankie with a ribbon. Other group members talked about different physically comforting habits they had: one slept with stuffed animals; another had a blanket.

Amal shared a story from when she was a child: on a family trip, her uncle asked if she and her two brothers wanted to go to McDonald's or Wendy's. Amal wanted Wendy's, but her brothers outnumbered her, so the family went to McDonald's. Amal refused to eat her burger. "There is nothing good about tantrumming," she said. "I was hungry and lonely and angry and left out!"

Ari asked Amal, "How does it feel to tantrum to us right now?"

Amal looked around the group. "It seems to be going okay!" Ari invited her to show more of her tantrumming side in the group.

In this example, group members were able to revisit their childhoods with the clear vision of adulthood. By noting the new, softer behavior of Catherine's fingers, I was able to help her remember the positive memory of soothing herself with a blanket, which led others to recall their own sources of early comfort. Amal remembered a pivotal experience from childhood that taught her that getting in touch with her angry feelings was bad and would leave her isolated and alone. In both cases, the past was integrated into the present in ways that opened new avenues for group members to relate to painful feelings.

As Ormont (2001) emphasizes, therapy groups can expand members' abilities to attract and sustain healthy relationships,

> In the hands of the skilled group analyst, the patient with intimacy problems has them evoked, can enact his defenses, can come to recognize his resistances, can work them through, and in the group can cultivate the ability to love and to experience love.

(p. 101)

References

Asplund, M., Rück, C., Lenhard, F., Gunnarsson, T., Bellander, M., Delby, H., & Ivanov, V. (2021). ACT-enhanced group behavior therapy for trichotillomania and skin-picking disorder: A feasibility study. *Journal of Clinical Psychology*, 77(7), 1537–1555.

Diefenbach, G., Tolin, D., Hannan, S., Maltby, N., & Crocetto, J. (2006). Group treatment for trichotillomania: Behavior therapy versus supportive therapy. *Behavior Therapy*, 37(4), 353–363.

Gulassa, D., Amaral, R., Oliviera, E., & Tavares, H. (2019). Group therapy for excoriation disorder: Psychodrama versus support therapy. *Annals of Clinical Psychiatry*, 31(2), 84–94.

Morris, J. (2021). Cinderella, the wicked queen, and Glinda walk into a group: Countertransference resistance and the group leader. In Y. Kane, S. Masselink, & A. Weiss (Eds.), *Women, intersectionality, and power in group therapy leadership* (pp. 108–122). New York, NY: Routledge.

Nakell, S. (2015). A healing herd: Benefits of a psychodynamic group approach in treating body-focused repetitive behaviors. *International Journal of Group Psychotherapy, 65*(11), 295–396.

Natterson-Horowitz, B., & Bowers, K. (2013). *Zoobiquity: The astonishing connection between human and animal health.* New York, NY: Vintage Books.

Neff, K. (2009). The role of self-compassion in development: A healthier way to relate to oneself. *Human Development, 52*(4), 211–214.

Ormont, L. R. (2001). *The technique of group treatment: The collected papers of Louis R. Ormont, Ph.D.* Furgeri, L. (Ed.). Madison, CT: Psychosocial Press.

Ragilienė, T. (2016). Links of adolescents identity development and relationship with peers: A systemic literature review. *Journal of the Canadian Academy of Child and Adolescent Psychiatry, 25*(2), 97–105.

Rosenthal, L. (1987). *Resolving resistance in group psychotherapy.* Northbale, NJ: Jason Aronson Inc.

Rosenthal, L. (1996). Phenomena of resistance in modern group analysis. *American Journal of Psychotherapy, 50*(1), 75–89.

Spotnitz, H., & Nagelberg, L. (1960). A preanalytic technique for resolving the narcissistic defense. *Psychiatry: Interpersonal and Biological Processes, 23*(2), 193–197.

Yalom, I., & Leszcz, M. (2020). *The theory and practice of group psychotherapy* (6th ed.). New York, NY: Basic Books.

8 Families in therapy
Healing the system

Family therapy for body-focused repetitive behaviors (BFRBs)

While I am not a family therapist by training, I have found that, because preteens and teens are still immersed in the family system, it makes sense to include the family in the treatment process to some extent. For those of you who want to better understand the theory and practice of family therapy from this perspective, I recommend Lewis' (2020) "Attachment-based family therapy for adolescent substance abuse: A move to the level of systems." The author describes a model called Behavior Exchange and Systems Therapy, which is designed to repair attachment disruptions and traumatic experiences within the family system.

Although books on family therapy are widely available, and a number of books have been written for parents of children with BFRBs, there are very few resources for therapists working with families with BFRBs. In 2000, Neziroglu et al. provided an overview of BFRB treatment for obsessive-compulsive disorder (OCD) and related disorders, including family therapy, behavioral and family therapy. The authors explained that family involvement in treatment does tend to positively affect treatment outcome for teens in therapy for disorders under the OCD umbrella, "Through incidental reporting and limited empiric data, the inclusion of the family in therapy enhances treatment outcome" (p. 660).

Keuthen et al. (2013) pointed out some of the stressors specific to teens with trichotillomania, including less freedom of emotional expression and higher levels of family conflict than their peers. In my work with teens and preteens, I have found that If I can help their parents shift the dynamic at home in some way that reduces the stressors that lead an adolescent to pick or pull, I can be much more effective with the adolescent. Because the behaviors are not deeply engrained at these ages, they can be much easier to treat. Sometimes in this age group people can

DOI: 10.4324/9781003299097-11

let go of negative behaviors altogether, though moderation remains our agreed-upon goal.

Neziroglu et al. (2000) pointed to a key element of work with families: once the family members understand the disorder, they can avoid blaming or punishing the teen for their reliance on BFRBs. One key to helping a family unit shift into a healing dynamic is to work with the parents on the shame they have felt since their child developed a very visible problem. I have found that parents almost universally wonder what they have done wrong. I introduce them to the resources at bfrb.org, which help them understand that they are not alone. It is important to acknowledge both that the family is in this together and that they have all been doing their best to cope with a difficult situation.

At the same time, I emphasize that the family is a system, and that it will help each person to reckon with the stresses that face them all. We will usually encounter a stressor in the whole family system that has been highlighted by the teen's BFRBD. This can include family conflict, divorce or a death in the family. These kinds of stressors will test any underlying difficulties with emotional regulation or communication within the family unit.

As we have explored, though they may be doing their best, if parents are taxed beyond their usual coping mechanisms without enough support, they won't be able to help their children grieve or process their emotions. Instead, painful feelings are often pushed aside, undigested and children in the family have no choice but to follow their parents' emotional lead.

Sometimes, I can help the family shift their perspective on the identified patient. Rather than acting badly or trying to cause problems, the sensitive child is bringing a gift of awareness to feelings that need to come out in the open.

The family in treatment

I include the parents in the treatment process from the start. Both they and their child fill out intake forms before we meet. I invite parents to the first session. This session allows each family member to share their view of why the client's picking and pulling developed, and how they have been handling it as a family since it became a problem. Everything about the way the family interacts, from where they choose to sit to how a parent responds if the child tears up within a session, helps me begin to understand their unique family system.

Usually, parents have in some way tried to fix the problem, by either insisting on various behavioral interventions or taking the child to see a therapist who focused on getting rid of the behavior or punishing the child when they pick or pull. Such situations do require some repair. In these intake sessions, the teen often is able to make a clear request of the parents to back off. I often frustrate parents when I support this request, letting them they can be most helpful by not mentioning the behaviors at all unless requested by the teen. This process works best if we can think of ourselves as a team, all working together to help with what has also become a family stressor, the BFRBD.

We make an important agreement about the teen's (a minor) confidentiality. We agree that my conversations with the teen will not be shared with the parents. If I have a concern about the teen's safety, I will first let them know that we need to tell their parents and give them the choice of either bringing parents into the session or me following up with them after. This first conversation sets us up to work as a team, a critical component of success when working with an adolescent.

Family sessions can empower parents to make changes in family dynamics that will in turn relieve pressure on the teen. Bringing unspoken concerns out into the open can unbottle long-contained feelings and not only help the teen let go of destructive behaviors but also help the family move forward.

Katelyn

My experience with Katelyn illustrates the ways that family therapy can support and enhance individual work with teenagers. Katelyn is a Caucasian female who came to see me for individual therapy for distress about pulling hair from her lashes and brows when she was 15. We worked together for 2 years, mostly in individual therapy with adjunct family support.

Katelyn displayed some of the usual characteristics of teens with BFRBDs. She was sensitive, both physiologically and emotionally. She experienced both depression and anxiety. Very bright, she was a student at a prestigious magnet school and could easily relate to the idea of perfectionism and over-achieving. She was mildly socially awkward but had a nice group of friends at school. She came to see me when her brows and lashes were visibly thin after a particularly stressful week of finals. Katelyn's people-pleasing defense had been very successful, and this crisis was the first major sign to her parents that her happy demeanor might not be the whole story.

When Katelyn came for an intake session with her parents, they all agreed that a family stressor was the demands her sister, 2 years younger, made on her parents, leaving less attention for Katelyn. Katelyn cried while leaning into her mom and agreed that she did feel like her needs came second to her sister's and that she wanted more from each of her parents. In that first session, they agreed to work on setting boundaries with her sister rather than just telling Katelyn that she's the older sister and should just be nice.

Katelyn felt neither of her parents fully understood her struggle with hair pulling. Her mom, as the primary caretaker, was the one who engaged more directly with her about her concern. As a result, she took most of the heat of

Katelyn's anger. This situation is common for primary caretakers, usually but of course not always female. The other parent is often the better liked parent but is less involved. It can be helpful for couples to address these dynamics through their own work. The more the parents can work together to share the process of helping their adolescent, the better. This was true in Katelyn's case. Because she and her mother experienced more conflict, it was her mother that we invited to follow-up sessions as needed with Dad supporting Mom.

In these sessions, we resolved some key conflicts between them. When Katelyn had first admitted to her mom that she pulled out her hair, her mom immediately focused on fixing the problem through behavioral strategies. The intervention made Katelyn furious and she had responded by pulling away emotionally. This feedback was hard for mother to hear, but with my help she was able to let herself off the hook. She let Katelyn know she was sorry and would take Katelyn's lead on behavioral strategies.

In her post-therapy interview, 3 months after we had completed our work together, Katelyn described that session as a pivotal moment, both in terms of her relationship with her mother and her own self-compassion about hair pulling.

> It was a lot easier once we were communicating. I told her that when she wanted me to put Band-Aids on all the time, she made me feel bad. I was judgmental toward myself, and once she agreed to back off, it just helped a lot.

In another session, Katelyn appreciated hearing more about her mother's own struggles. "All the sudden, a bunch of things made sense. Like, why she did certain things that she did or why she was acting the way she acted. Knowing she's had some of the struggles that I have is helpful."

By the time she left treatment, Katelyn's hair pulling had almost fully resolved. She credits this shift to finding her own favorite fiddles and learning to regulate her emotions.

> I always have something to mess with, and now it's more automatic where I get that feeling and I'm like . . . I should pick up a pencil or something. A lot of it was understanding my emotions, because then it just got easier to sort of explain, this is upsetting me and we should do something about this.

Colt

Colt's case, featured in a case review in Dermatologic Therapy (Aukerman et al., 2021) was more complicated. Colt had experienced medical trauma at a very early age, and his life and that of his young parents had revolved around his care for the first 8 years of his life. We worked together for 15 months, in a combination of individual and family therapy. At the end of that time, Colt had let go of his hair-pulling behavior, and his gains were maintained at the time of our 6-month post-therapy interview and a 5 year follow-up.

Colt had been born with a spinal imbalance. The surgeries to correct the imbalance were largely successful, but they had left him with some physical, cognitive and learning issues. These included a unique, higher pitched voice and difficulties with sensory processing. Since the age of 4 or 5, he had gone through a range of fidgety behaviors that were deeply annoying to his parents, including excessively tucking in his shirts and picking at his fingers, before he discovered, after a bout with lice at the age of 11, that pulling out his hair felt good. He then developed trichotillomania, or, as he called it, "playing with my hair."

Colt's hair pulling was automatic. His hands were in his hair, feeling, finding and pulling, for hours and hours at a time, whether in front of the TV or riding in a car or even in class during a test. When he pulled his hair at home, his parents would gently bring his attention to what he was doing, and his hands would go down, only to head right back up to his scalp. He had developed bald spots and had to get permission to wear a baseball cap to school after a bullying incident. His parents sought my services when they realized they were at their wits' end and didn't know how to help their son.

As I explained in Chapter 5, we usually get through the safety phase before delving into trauma histories. In Colt's case, to my surprise, we did a key piece of trauma work in our first session. When I reflected on that moment, I realized that an important part of his experience had been building up in him without words for a very long time.

I remember Colt's mother telling me in our first phone conversation that I would fall in love with him. She was right, and I felt connected to him from the moment we met. It wasn't that we skipped the safety phase; it was that Colt assessed my office quickly, and once he felt it was safe enough, the story burst out of him.

At 11, Colt was sweet, bouncy and full of personality. When he came into my office, Colt looked around at all the items I had lying around and the various chairs I had in place for the family session. He settled himself onto the couch, put the blanket over himself and picked out a pillow to go under his head and a caterpillar fiddle toy from the fiddle tray. He said, "Hi, I'm Colt." His parents sat down, and our relationship began.

I asked his parents a few questions about Colt's life, while Colt stayed quiet as his fingers explored the textures of the items he had chosen. His mother briefly mentioned his numerous surgeries and noted that they had been blessed with family support and good medical care. They talked about Colt's long history of repetitive behaviors and reflected that he had never really been able to keep his hands still. When I asked the family why they thought he had developed these tics at an early age, they were at a loss.

I referenced his history of surgeries and suggested that sometimes bodies hold onto the effect of surgeries even if they leave no conscious memories. Colt immediately sat up and started talking. He told us that he had woken up through the anesthesia and remembered that he wasn't in pain but was terrified. He had never before spoken those words, and his parents had no idea that he had experienced that trauma. We all agreed it made sense that he hadn't had words for the experience before, because he was unable to access words at the moment under anesthesia. His parents validated and supported him as he cried while wrapping the blanket around himself. As they hugged him from either side, I felt a palpable sense of relief in the room.

Colt and I met weekly for 15 months. As usual, I was flexible about what combination of family and individual therapy would be most helpful. We gave him the choice of how long his parents would be with us each session. He usually wanted them to come to the first half of each session, and then he would ask them to leave for the second half.

Initially, it was clear that spending time with his family in the room helped Colt to relax and build more trust in me. He would look at them frequently. In addition, he continued to want the room to be organized according to his preferences, and now had places where he wanted us each to sit. He snuggled up in the comfy blanket on the couch, occasionally putting his face under the blanket to indicate some embarrassment or need to pause. Later in therapy, he would ask them to leave sooner and sooner, and he opened up to me more and more.

Being in charge of the sessions gave Colt the sense of control he needed to counter the many times he had been powerless early in his life. This dynamic was key to our success. His mom reflected, "He had his own preparation for each session. He would take his shoes off, arrange himself in the blanket, get the red caterpillar. He could take control of whatever made him comfortable."

Colt's baseball cap became the subject of an important behavioral intervention in our work. The cap had been helpful to Colt through the fifth grade, as it built his confidence and helped him sidestep some of the bullying that had been directed toward him. By the end of that school year, however, his parents were beginning to wonder if it was also becoming a crutch, allowing him to continue the behavior without facing its consequences. I saw their point, and so did Colt, if reluctantly.

We agreed to take the summer to focus on reducing his hair-pulling behaviors, including addressing his impulsivity and finding sensory replacements.

His mom noticed that Colt liked to pick the fluff off his socks during our sessions, and he expanded his range of calming behaviors to include less destructive options.

In the family part of our sessions, Colt's parents often brought up issues or conflicts that Colt might not have mentioned on his own. Colt and I used those concerns as a jumping-off point for our conversations when we were alone. In addition to hair pulling, Colt struggled with other impulsive behaviors, getting into verbal conflicts with friends and having overblown tantrums at home. I helped him to put into words the feelings that lay deeper than the impulses.

The first step in helping Colt to regulate his emotions was to help him pay attention to and understand what he was feeling. I noticed that when he talked about math class or math tutoring, his hand would often go straight to his hair, and he was able to translate that to the nervousness he felt about failing and disappointing his parents. Once he talked about the nervousness, his hand didn't seem to need to go back to his hair. In his words, "Stacy taught me how to deal with the nervous stuff. When I was coming here, my hair pulling was out of control. But then when I left, I was totally controlled."

We discovered that Colt's stress cup was full or even overflowing with frustration about how hard things could be for him compared to other kids his age. When he was picked on, he would become immediately enraged, lashing out physically and getting in trouble at school. Breath work helped him to engage his parasympathetic nervous system and gave him some time to make a different choice. He hated being called to the principal's office and was very receptive to working on assertiveness skills to replace lashing out. Colt especially enjoyed role playing with me as the bully, looking me straight in the eye and telling me to back off and leave him alone. This helped him to effectively tell a friend to back off ribbing him at school.

Colt returned to his medical history only once more, a couple of months into our work, when memories were triggered by a trip to the emergency room. A fall had left him needing stitches, and he had a very hard time with the experience, screaming, crying and pulling at his hair during the procedure. We talked about the parts of the experience that reminded him of his earlier surgeries, including not being able to stop what was happening, and I validated for him that it must have been almost impossible to calm down while it was happening. We talked about how he had gotten through it, and that it was safe to calm down now. We worked on deep belly breathing together and he was able to relax.

The other key piece of our work was to resolve the trauma Colt's parents had experienced. Ten months into treatment, Colt's mother expressed her utter frustration with Colt's fairly typical teenage behaviors, and I invited her to come in for a session. It was our first session alone, and she was able to let down the strong front she had maintained for years. She cried as she talked about what it was like for her to go through those terrifying surgeries with her newborn, and the many losses and sacrifices she experienced along the way. In a session with both parents, Colt's dad was able to acknowledge his own pain, and, though he wasn't as openly emotional as his wife, was able to comfort her. They realized that they didn't need to react to every rebellious comment Colt might make at home and gave him more space to be frustrated and uncooperative.

A few weeks before sixth grade was to begin, Colt and I revisited our goal of leaving the baseball cap at home. Colt felt happy about the short hairs that had grown in over the summer as he pulled less and less, and we agreed that a buzz cut would give him a fresh start for the school year. Soon after, he decided he was ready to leave therapy.

Colt's dad noted the importance of my relationship with Colt to the success of the work: "He was totally comfortable being with her and they were so happy to see each other all of the time." Dad added that my relationship with both parents was equally important: "I think the relationship with Stacy evolved. When we first came, it was all about Colt, and then it became about this family working really hard. She joined in that fight with us."

Colt himself described our work as transformative, both in allowing him to let go of hair pulling and in seeing himself differently: "I feel better about myself, which made me stop playing with my hair. That is one thing I conquered. I nailed it." His mom agreed and assessed their success as a family: "I feel like we all conquered it."

Team approach

For my work with preteens and teens, I have come to understand that a team approach is usually necessary to help them through the adolescent years. With a deficit of skills to cope with the particularly fraught world of grade school, they greatly benefit from group or intensive outpatient programs focusing on skill-building. Dialectical behavior therapy (DBT) is particularly helpful with this age group. With body dysmorphic disorder a common comorbid condition, eating issues also go hand in hand with BFRBs in adolescence, and often a nutritionist is part of the team. In addition, underlying depression and anxiety should be assessed by a doctor, psychiatrist or psychiatric nurse practitioner. While medications can be useful, they also must be used with special care. I have found that it is helpful to let the whole family know that as the adolescent begins to assert their needs through our work, they often enter a time of expected conflict with parents.

Often an outside family therapist is important part of the team. For many teens, having a therapist other than me to work with the family is preferable, as they prefer to keep me as their personal resource.

Barriers to success

Of course, it is natural for families to feel anxious and reluctant about giving family therapy a try. Some parents insist that the disorder is a behavioral problem that has nothing to do with them as a family, and it is not possible to form a team with them. Sometimes I connect parents to other providers for family therapy, and positive changes happen in the family dynamic. Individual work with adolescents without family buy-in is usually less successful but can still be helpful.

One factor that is important to remember about working with adolescents is that this is a time when they are pushing hard against their parents. It is natural for parents to feel some sadness and envy when they see their emotionally inaccessible teen sharing their feelings with a therapist. It is important for parents to understand that pulling away is one part of the developmental process for teens, and we can help connect parents to more support as needed to cope with this difficult process.

Cultural expectations must be taken into account in family treatment, and they present their own set of challenges, demanding cultural humility from the therapist. For example, a first-generation Indian American family came to me with the expectation that I would fix their daughter's hair pulling before they visited India later in the year. The daughter, struggling to navigate the mix of Indian and American cultures in adolescence, stubbornly resisted that deadline. My work was complicated by the need to respect and validate both perspectives, and my errors on one side or another along the way. In the end, I worked with the teen for a full year, and we all agreed she had gained a lot from our sessions, though they also expressed their frustration with her lack of behavioral progress.

Each family comes to therapy with a unique mix of stressors and strengths. In working with families, it is key to maintain flexibility and be responsive to each family dynamic.

References

Aukerman, E., Nakell, S., & Jafferany, M. (2021). Psychodynamic approach in the treatment of trichotillomania. *Dermatologic Therapy*. DOI:10.1111/dth.15218

Keuthen, N., Fama, J., Altenburger, E., Allen, A., Raff, A., & Pauls, D. (2013). Family environment in adolescent trichotillomania. *Journal of Obsessive-Compulsive and Related Disorders*, 2(4), 366–374.

Lewis, A. (2020). Attachment-based family therapy for adolescent substance use: A move to the level of systems. *Frontiers of Psychiatry*. https://doi.org/10.3389/fpsyt.2019.00948

Neziroglu, F., Hsia, C., & Yaryura-Tobias, J. (2000). Behavioral, cognitive and family therapy for obsessive-compulsive and related disorders. *Psychiatric Clinics of North America, 23*(3), 657–670.

9   Moving into maintenance or ending treatment

Bittersweet goodbyes

In therapy, as in life, saying goodbye is a difficult task. Goodbyes bring up each client's (and therapist's!) former losses and partings, tendencies to leave without resolving ruptures in the relationship, and impulses to bolt when strong feelings arise. Cognitive-behavioral treatment usually ends when the goal of symptom resolution is achieved, perhaps as indicated on a questionnaire or through clients' self-reporting. From a psychodynamic perspective, the process of concluding treatment is more nuanced. Creating healthy treatment endings is an important task in my work. If I can facilitate goodbyes that are honest, reflective and relational, I can help each client learn how to enact healthier goodbyes with others in their lives.

Of course, this is easier said than done. When a client leaves without talking through the reasons for the departure, and before agreed-upon goals have been met, that's a negative treatment outcome. This kind of ending leaves both parties feeling incomplete. The therapist doesn't get the opportunity to understand what happened to cause the sudden departure, and any relationship wounds harbored by the client don't get tended to or repaired. Although premature terminations do happen to all therapists, they can be greatly mitigated, in my experience, through the psychodynamic approach.

A healthy ending includes a mutual review between client and therapist of goals that have been achieved, how they were achieved, and what tools the clients can carry with them into the future, when new challenges arise. These are goals agreed upon during the safety phase of therapy. They include building emotional regulation and communication and assertiveness skills, improving relationships, and meeting life goals such as finding a healthy relationship or parenting effectively.

When a client suggests that they may be ready to leave individual or group therapy, we assess: are we really done with our work, or is this a

DOI: 10.4324/9781003299097-12

distress signal about something unresolved that we need to put into words? Do they have the coping skills they need to avoid a painful relapse of symptoms when new challenges arise, or are they impatient to "graduate" from therapy? Are they more at peace with themselves as hair pullers or skin pickers? Have they befriended painful emotions, such as anger and sadness? And, importantly, have they developed or enhanced a supportive community in which they can utilize communication skills and in which their feelings are welcomed? If they decide to leave, we figure out how many more sessions they would like for the closure process – usually from one to three for individual work, or 3 weeks for group work.

Some clients choose to continue in therapy on a long-term basis after meeting initial goals, to continue to develop and maintain healthy relationships. In this chapter, I will explore some of the complexities of each of these types of endings: premature, healthy and maintenance.

Early termination

Early termination is a recurring problem for many cognitive-behavioral therapists, making up 40% of the endings in CBT for depression (Leahy, 2001). Research hasn't focused on premature terminations with the BFRBD population; however, the frequency of relapses and cross-addictions is a sign that CBT treatment hasn't helped the majority of clients find sustainable alternatives to their problematic behaviors. Unfortunately, BFRB relapses bring more shame, and for perfectionists that often lead to a downward spiral. Someone who has ended CBT treatment as a "success" is not likely to return after experiencing what they can see as only failure. A negative therapy experience may discourage clients from seeking help again.

Robert Leahy (2001), a cognitive-behavioral therapist, provides some insight into relapses. He explains that a weakness of CBT is the rigid focus on symptoms and structured treatment packages. A passionate believer in CBT, he explains how a wider and deeper case conceptualization can reduce the factors that lead to early termination. He emphasizes that case formulation must include attention to the psychosocial complexities of each individual, such as choice of relationships, coping strategies, and beliefs about the self and others. He clarifies that these underlying issues will lead to resistance to behavioral change if left unaddressed.

Healthy endings

In a review of the literature on premature termination, Swift et al. (2012) note that up to 20% of clients end treatment prematurely regardless of the therapist's theoretical stance. The authors described six factors that can reduce early endings: educating clients about duration of treatment and patterns of change, clarifying the roles of therapist and client, incorporating each client's individual preferences into the treatment, strengthening early hope, fostering the therapeutic alliance and routinely discussing the treatment to assess how the process is going.

Bhatia & Gelso (2017) make clear that a healthy ending process is key to the overall success of a therapeutic relationship.

> A central message of the present study seems to be for therapists to consider how clients are experiencing the termination phase and the therapeutic relationship components during the termination phase, as the working alliance, real relationship, and negative transference during the termination phase are associated with successful termination work. An effective termination phase in turn, appears to be associated with better overall treatment outcomes.
>
> (p. 86)

I weave many of these conditions into the integrative psychodynamic treatment I have outlined throughout this book. The safety phase is important in setting the stage for the conditions of success as we move through a comprehensive assessment, educate our clients about the process of therapy, co-create goals and build a therapeutic alliance. Our work has established the atmosphere for the co-regulation of emotions, and healing goes deeper than behavioral change to improve the client's relationships and quality of life.

I rarely experience early terminations. In my practice, about two-thirds of clients adjourn in a healthy way, while the remaining third stay with me for maintenance treatment. In my experience, those who have a stronger support network in their lives are those most likely to adjourn from treatment, while those for whom I have become an important attachment figure may choose to continue.

Both outcomes – adjourning and continuing – are healthy, led by the client's needs, and discussed together. A healthy ending can itself be a corrective emotional experience, as saying goodbye with integrity and connection is an important skill to learn, and one my clients have rarely experienced. While I usually let the client bring up the topic of ending our work together, there are times when I notice a client pulling away from therapy, such as arriving late or seeming uninterested in talking to me, and I will check in to see how they are feeling about therapy and whether there are thoughts of departure. In the following paragraphs, I will share a few client endings.

Adjourning

Around 4 months into our work together, Anna, whom you may remember from Chapter 6, suggested that she might be ready to end treatment. When I asked Anna about her motivation to leave therapy, she talked about being mad at me for opening up so many feelings inside of her without fixing them or making them go away. At that point, her skin-picking behaviors were continuing and even increasing in intensity. She was also more uncomfortable about the "picking binges" (her words) because she was more aware of them.

While noting that I would respect her decision to leave when the right time came, I wondered aloud if we might be in the very kind of moment we had talked about in our initial session, when she was experiencing discomfort in our work together and wanted to get away from those feelings.

I suggested that if we let the process unfold a bit more, she would be able to get closer to the goals we had set together – to rely less on her picking behaviors, to understand the triggers that set them in motion and to be kinder to herself when she does pick her skin.

In her 3-month post-treatment interview, she reflected that she was glad I had challenged her to determine what she might be running away from. She realized that her anger at me and frustration with the process had led her to want to leave therapy:

> At first, being in a truly nonjudgmental environment where someone truly understands you and wants to help you is, like, freeing! But then, also, there was a large quantity of emotional baggage to get out and I was frustrated, and I told Stacy!
>
> That was partly my desire to finish therapy, to conquer my skin picking, though I realized through the course of it that it was not totally the goal. Sometimes, I didn't want to come. Just the feeling of having to go and feel this again. Sometimes, it's like you just don't want to.

This moment was an example of how resistance to feeling painful feelings can lead to early termination, and how it doesn't have to. Anna agreed to continue treatment, and we continued weekly for 2 more months. During that time, she started to implement some of the new behaviors we worked on, such as asking her husband more often to watch the children so that she could take a minute of rest for herself instead of sneaking into the bathroom to pick her skin.

After 2 months, she again brought up the idea of ending treatment, this time with a different motive: "I wanted to see what it would feel like to just take some of the lessons I learned in therapy and let them sink in." Now, as we reflected on her progress together, we agreed that she had met her goals. In her post-treatment interview, she explained,

> I feel like I'm in control of my life and my picking and I've let go of the garbage and guilt behind it. Probably the most helpful part was digging up all of those old episodes in different parts of my life and how I used picking to cope. I am just nicer to myself.

She also pointed out that therapy didn't have a perfect ending, as she still sometimes finds herself in a "deep picking tunnel": "The difference is that most days don't feel like that, and I can remind myself that picking is still a way I use to cope with stressors, just not as often." She utilizes a number of other healthy coping methods to redirect those feelings.

Adjournment session

The final session itself serves an important role – honoring our work together and reaffirming new coping skills. A recent adjournment session with a teen, Mary, captured that flow.

Mary is a Caucasian female who came to see me at 15 for hair pulling and anxiety. Two years into our biweekly work together, she told me she thought she was ready to leave treatment. She said that she understood why she pulls and has managed to reduce pulling from her eyelashes and brows enough to keep from feeling self-conscious. Both of her parents were a bit anxious about her ending treatment while she still engaged in some hair pulling, and we agreed to move our meetings to once a month for 2 months to make sure she felt ready to go.

At our final session, Mary was clear: she was ready to end our work together. We spoke about her progress toward the goals we had set together and the ways she felt more able to regulate her emotions on her own. I asked her what had changed in her relationships that had helped her to cope with the stresses of COVID-19 quarantine during the 2020 school year without increasing her pulling. "I open up!" she said. "I get things off of my chest earlier now, so they don't fill up my stress cup and lead me to pulling as intensely."

As we reviewed our time together, I brought up a session from around a year earlier, one that I thought had led to a lot of growth on her part. At that session, Mary had admitted to holding a grudge against me from the beginning of our work, because I had never followed up about some experiences with suicidal friends that she had mentioned early on. Once she had voiced her frustration, we had talked through these experiences, and eventually her anxiety about death abated to some extent. Now, she reflected on why I might have flagged that particular session as pivotal: "You liked it that I was so assertive, and then I got what I needed from you."

We looked ahead at Mary's plans for coping with life stressors without falling back on her hair-pulling behaviors and starting the cycle over again. As she had pointed out many times, it's very hard to grow backlashes and brows, and devastatingly easy to pull them all out. During a recent stressful experience – writing a college essay – she noticed herself tugging on her lashes, the first step of her pulling trance. She caught herself and picked up her putty, her favorite fiddle toy, and kneaded it to get some of the frustration out.

We agreed that having fiddle toys in her most likely picking environments, including her computer desk, was key. Her sense was that the putty could be soothing enough to keep her present and focused on her essays for the next couple of days. She also mentioned that as long as she kept slip-ups in perspective and didn't make a big deal about them, she could now usually keep them from turning into relapses.

As we finished the review of our relationship, Mary wondered if she would ever let go of hair pulling completely. I reminded her that the research shows teens and preteens are the most likely to be able to leave BFRBs behind, integrating more mature coping mechanisms as they move into adulthood. Reassured, she said goodbye.

In her 3-month post-treatment interview, Mary explained that she ended treatment because she no longer needed me:

> It started to be like, even if something bad happened, it wasn't something that I couldn't handle, and now I talk more about my feelings with my friends. The hair pulling is way less frequent or intense, and between putty, putting on and picking off nail polish, and petting my cats, I have things I can do with my hands instead of pulling.

Mixed adjournment and continuation

Sometimes, one type of treatment ends but another continues. Elise, from Chapter 7, was the last founding member to leave the group in the case study. She had joined the group after several years in individual treatment with me and continued biweekly throughout. As the group diversified beyond the early mix of Caucasian young adult females, Elise was able to work more directly on developing intimacy with men and on sharing her struggle with skin picking with others.

Initially, Elise had been the only skin picker alongside a number of hair pullers. Elise had expressed annoyance about that fact and noted that she was the "messiest" of the bunch, with less perfect hair, clothes and image.

She was also the likeliest to get angry while the others were more likely to express sadness. She hoped another skin picker would join the group.

To my surprise, when I did bring in another member who picked her skin, Elise found the connection too close for comfort. At that point, after being in the group for 5 years, Elise had met many of her life goals. She had married a nice man, established boundaries with her family of origin and was able to share more of her feelings in her relationships outside of the group therapy room. While her skin picking continued, it was less intense and no longer interfered with her life in the ways it had before.

Despite her own struggles with BFRBs, Elise struggled to empathize with the new member, who was much deeper in her skin-picking struggle. Only a couple of weeks after the new member joined, Elise decided that she would leave the group. I was disappointed that she wasn't interested in exploring her negative feelings toward the new member. She said she needed to focus on herself, as she was starting infertility treatments. In this case, I had to process my own countertransference reaction so as not to let my disappointment get in the way of letting her leave the group.

Elise had a healthy goodbye process with the group, with three closure sessions, as agreed in the contract. She left the group feeling empowered by the process of choosing where to invest her energy and decided to continue in maintenance individual treatment with me.

In her 3-month post-group interview, she talked about the benefits of her participation in the group.

As she put it,

> When I first came to Stacy, I explained picking as kind of like running a news ticker on the bottom screen of bad news and bad thoughts, and kind of watching that screen and being in a trance. Whereas now, I'm way more aware of what I'm doing.

This mindfulness didn't lead to a decrease in frequency of picking for Elise, but it did reduce the shame associated with it, as well as the intensity of damage done. Elise was able to see increases in picking as a signal to check in with what she was feeling, rather than as a failing.

Group therapy also helped Elise form and maintain better social and intimate connections. She learned to navigate conflicts by talking about her feelings rather than exploding and was able to empathize with others even during disagreements. In her words,

> In group, it's like taking a step back and seeing the bigger picture, and not just acting out the usual pattern. I've noticed that when I get angry

now, I pull back from my usual furious responses, and can put myself in the other person's shoes.

Her experience talking about skin picking in the group went well enough that she brought others in her life into her inner circle, sharing her vulnerabilities rather than hiding them. She was also influenced by seeing another member suffer the toll of suppressing emotions. This led Elise to nurture deeper connections, which ultimately helped her find a loving partner.

As I write this, Elise and I continue individual therapy. At first we focused on her struggles with infertility, and now on her transition to life as a new mother. While at the time I expected her to remain in the group when she decided to leave, over time I have understood how important it was for her to be able to leave group treatment behind to focus only on her own needs in therapy.

Maintenance treatment

Like Elise, some clients, especially those who do not have a nurturing relationship with some or all members of their family of origin, choose to remain in therapy long term, sometimes with decreased frequency, as an important continuation of care. In this period, although many goals may have been met, we work to build complex adaptive emotional regulation skills such as communication, allowing vulnerability and assertiveness. In addition, the healthy attachment between the therapist and client facilitates the maintenance of treatment gains. The image that comes to mind with these ongoing relationships is me as a stake in the ground on which my clients, like individual tomato vines, can grow and expand securely.

We met Andi, a Caucasian female, in Chapter 4. She sought treatment for trichotillomania and trichophagia when she was 26 years old, and we met weekly for many years. Several years into our work, she decided to shift to seeing me monthly. Altogether, Andi and I have been working together for 12 years.

When she first came to see me, Andi was in great distress about her secret engagement in pulling out and eating her hair. She found the hair eating in particular so disgusting that she decided in my office, at our first session, not to do it again. We were, of course, only in the safety phase. I was clear with her about my reluctance to get on board with that plan, as it might set us up for failure. I told her about the risk of cross-addictions, and she decided she would rather overeat or pick at her skin (her other go-to comforts) than pull and eat her hair. And she actually did almost completely stop that behavior from that moment on.

As I got to know Andi, I began to understand why she needed our work together to demarcate a before and an after in her identity as a hair puller.

Ever since pulling her first hair at the age of 10, she had labeled the part of herself that pulls and eats hair as not only bad but monstrous, and her hair itself as disgusting. She needed to shed that identity in order to allow self-compassion to build. Andi reflected on that shift:

> From our initial contact, I felt very comfortable and cared for by Stacy. But it took a while to realize that there was no compassion for myself. It took even longer to build that compassion, to where now I can talk to myself, like, it's going to be OK. I brush my hair with love now, I really started loving my hair, and recognizing that it is really beautiful, and I can take care of it and be nicer to myself.

Another main task for our work was for Andi to identify her feelings, especially anger, and to learn that she could express those feelings without losing relationships. She explains,

> I feel like I was always angry at my mom and there was no room for me to have anger with her, I guess. But I'm learning in therapy that relationships possibly can withstand different emotions, including anger. And the pulling, and chewing, [which] I used to push my feelings down, I don't need them as much.

Over the years, Andi's life changed and lightened. She shed parts of her life that had been holding her back. This included getting a divorce from an unhappy marriage, marrying a kind man and getting a very good, high-powered job in a field she loved. She has continued to engage in some skin-picking and overeating behaviors, but at a level that doesn't cause much distress. She had never been interested in joining one of my groups, and at some point, our individual work started to feel different. She was doing very well, and there was a shift in how much she needed from me. It was at that point that she asked if we could move from weekly to monthly sessions.

As we reflected on why she chose that option rather than adjourning, she told me that talking about her feelings keeps the urge to pull out her hair from building too high, and she does still have these urges from time to time. She considered our time together as the key to coping with the stresses of work and the ways that negative self-talk could take over if she made any mistakes. In her interview, she explained,

> There's still things that come up in my relationships, and continuing therapy helps me understand where those feelings are coming from and kind of work through those. I guess I'm still learning and I feel like I have more work to do.

Although she has managed to have a relationship with both of her parents, they do not provide the kind of comfort and support she gets from me. She was emotional about the impact of our work:

> I'm just grateful. It has changed the course of my life, and I just think it's been a very good experience for me. And I'm fortunate enough at this point in my life that I can afford to continue. It's been a long time. Yeah. But I'd do it all over again.

References

Bhatia, A., & Gelso, C. (2017). The termination phase: Therapists' perspective on the therapeutic relationship and outcome. *Psychotherapy Research Practice Training, 54*, 76–87.

Leahy, R. (2001). *Overcoming resistance in cognitive therapy*. New York, NY: Guilford Press.

Swift, J., Greenberg, P., Whipple, J., & Kominiak, N. (2012). Practice recommendations for reducing premature terminations in therapy. *Professional Psychology: Research and Practice, 43*(4), 379–387.

Appendices

Appendix 1
Psychodynamic assessment

The assessment process is relational and ongoing, and we track as much of each client's life experience as possible. This worksheet outlines assessment categories that can help guide you through the process.

BFRB engagement

- Picking, pulling, biting, a combination?
- Intensity and negative consequences
- Frequency and duration
- Any idea about what triggers the behaviors?
- Other coping behaviors? (drugs, alcohol, food, sex)

Comorbid conditions

- Inquire about current medications and diagnoses by psychiatrists or past therapists
- Common conditions: depression, anxiety, body dysmorphic disorder, post-traumatic stress disorder, attention-deficit disorder with hyperactivity, obsessive-compulsive disorder
- Also consider non-clinical diagnoses that reflect normal reactions to immensely stressful circumstances, like Odysseus syndrome after traumatic migration experiences (Bianucci et al., 2017)

Precipitating factors

- When was the first occurrence of the behavior? What was going on in the psychosocial environment at that time?
- Make note of losses, unresolved grief and trauma

- Did perfectionism play a role?
- Was performance at school a factor?

Current triggers

- Places (car, school, bathroom, bed)
- Emotions (includes excitement, anger, fear)
- Psychosocial stressors (work, family, discrimination, poverty)
- Self-report and notice in session if hand goes to pick or pull

Dissociation

- Look for client signals – glazed eyes, losing train of thought, looking up a lot
- Notice countertransference – feeling dizzy, feeling floaty or losing train of thought. Mention the feeling and ask if the client also feels it
- Take the client's cue about whether they want to know more about dissociation, whether they want to name any trauma they have experienced
- Ground in the five senses: what do you hear, see, feel, taste, touch right not at the moment?
- Could also use the Dissociative Experiences Scale (Carlson & Putnam, 1993).

Level of shame/self-compassion

- How angry is the client at themselves for engaging in the behavior?
- Do they describe it with disgust?
- Do they see it as a coping strategy?

Marginalized identities

- It is important to find out how each client self-identifies race, sexual orientation and gender identity. Asking open questions and avoiding making assumptions are key.
- We may need to ask if we want to know how racism, sexism, homophobia or transphobia (among others) has affected our client's lives.
- We may need to ask to find out the impact our own identity has on our client, whether in similarities or differences (Comas-Díaz & Jacobsen, 1991).

- Remember that intersections of various marginalized identities can increase the stressors that trigger BFRBs.

References

Bianucci, R., Charlier, P., Perciaccante, A., Lippi, D., & Appenzeller, O. (2017). The "ulysses syndrome": An eponym identifies a psychosomatic disorder in modern migrants. *European Journal of Internal Medicine, 41*, 30–32.

Carlson, E., & Putnam, F. (1993). An update on the dissociative experiences scale. *Dissociation: Progress in the Dissociative Disorders, 6*(1), 16–27.

Comas-Díaz, L., & Jacobson, F. (1991). Ethnocultural transference and counter-transference in the therapeutic dyad. *American Journal of Orthopsychiatry, 61*(3), 692–402.

Appendix 2

Goals: behavioral, adaptive emotional regulation skills, improved quality of life

Goal-setting

Agreeing on goals is a key component of building a therapeutic alliance. Key question: what would success look like?

If the answer is, "No picking or pulling ever again," we need to shift expectations toward realistic goals.

Behavioral

- Harm reduction model, what level of picking or pulling could you live with without much distress?
- Allow for ups and downs in picking and pulling in reaction to life's stressors.
- Find the replacement fidgets that best meet individual sensory needs.

Adaptive emotional regulation skills

- Deep belly breathing, body awareness
- Awareness and tolerance of feelings
- Self-kindness
- Emotional expression
- Modulation of emotions
- Assertiveness
- Sublimation
- Healthy grooming/soft comforts

Enhanced quality of life

- Relationship goals
- Financial goals
- Familial goals
- Professional goals
- Existential-facing losses and disappointment

Appendix 3
Building self-compassion

Building self-compassion

Self-compassion has three components: mindfulness, self-kindness and a sense of universality (Neff, 2009). It can serve as an antidote to toxic shame. Psychoeducation can be a helpful tool in building self-compassion. First and foremost, it is important to see BFRBs as coping mechanisms rather than as problems. Once we accept their role, they are more likely to loosen their grip.

Psychoeducation

- Talk about how common BFRBs are; include info about the oral and other sensory elements that can be a part of it-bring in universality.
- Introduce the idea of self-compassion; explain that it can be an antidote to shame.
- Talk about the shame cycle and how hating a behavior can actually increase it.
- Introduce the idea of picking, pulling and biting as coping mechanisms; explain that this means even though the behaviors have felt like enemies, they were trying to help bring in self-kindness.
- Explain the sensory processing issues that usually underlie BFRBs, and note that it is just a bit harder for this population, "fiddlers," to soothe their central nervous systems. Need extra help, sensory replacements.

Mindfulness tools

- Breath work, in session and outside session, taking deep belly breaths

- Gentle body awareness, with the breath, where do you feel the breath coming in, what do you notice when it fills your chest (be aware that painful feelings may arise)
- Leads toward mentalization, the ability to notice what is happening inside of oneself while it is happening, develop a witness self, modulate emotions

Metaphor of the stress cup

- I like to think about a cup inside of each of us that is filled with our various stressors.
- When our stress cup is very full, urges will be impossible to resist, so we need to be compassionate with ourselves when we engage in BFRBs.
- When our stress cup is less full, due to reducing the stressors in our lives and/or developing better ways to get stress out of the body, the urges will be less strong and we have more of a choice whether to engage.
- Can we think more about reducing/expelling the stress that fills our cups and our body than trying to stop or resist body-focused behaviors?

Animal studies facts

- Animals also engage in body-focused behaviors, like a horse biting its flank. They do not engage in these behaviors in the wild. They do it when they enter the stressful environments of humans. Just like us, they get restless!
- Triggers for BFRBs in animals have been found: lack of sufficient space, isolation, boredom, frustration. Adding another animal to the mix, increasing pen size or allowing more grazing time can ameliorate the behaviors (Natterson-Horowitz & Bowers, 2013).
- How does each client relate to these triggers?
- What environmental changes might be able to ameliorate each client's BFRB?

References

Natterson-Horowitz, B., & Bowers, K. (2013). *Zoobiquity: The astonishing connection between human and animal health.* New York, NY: Vintage Books.

Neff, K. (2009). The role of self-compassion in development: A healthier way to relate to oneself. *Human Development, 52*(4), 211–214.

Appendix 4

Keys to the unconscious

Keys to the unconscious

I find a whiteboard to be the perfect vehicle for allowing the left brain to relax as the right brain allows unconscious material into the therapy room. In addition to mind-mapping, sometimes an image a client has in session will perk up my interest, and I'll grab the board and write. We make connections together as we go.

Mind-mapping

In this process, we start with one image or idea, and I draw lines to connect other images that come to mind. Often we learn something we wouldn't otherwise have learned.

Journal prompts/art prompts

- Create individualized suggestions to explore a metaphor or image or memory that arises during a session.
- Some people respond well to suggestions for between sessions "homework," and others prefer to leave the session at the door when they leave.

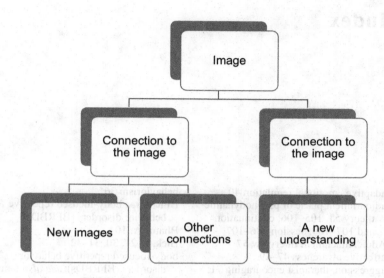

Figure A.1 An example of mind-mapping.

Index

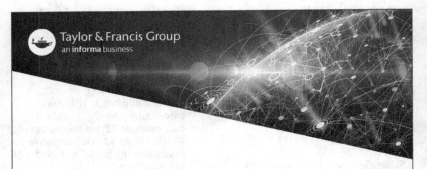

Printed in the United States
by Baker & Taylor Publisher Services